# Praise for Natalia Rose and The Raw Food Detox Diet (a.k.a. The Rose Program)

I feel so grateful for this program. I feel "enlightened," more energized, happier (I think people don't fully realize that what they eat can affect their moods), and finally for the first time in my life, I feel a greater sense of control regarding my eating habits. I've also experienced tremendous improvement with my asthmatic/allergy condition. I am no longer dependent on asthma medication. I am able to run five miles per day and have recently completed a half marathon! Like many, I've been a yo-yo dieter. Bottom line: I feel so much more "alive." Thank you, Natalia!

—*Danielle Reda*

I am so excited to be able to offer Natalia's extraordinary health and weight loss program at Radu Physical Culture. I highly recommend the program to anyone who has ever struggled with their weight or their health. It's both an education and a really fun journey. Once you go on this journey with her, your perception of food will be changed forever and you will never look back!

—*Radu, founder of the Radu*
*Physical Culture Gym in New York City*

It has been two and a half months since I've been working with Natalia and I have lost a total of 30 pounds and I'm continuing to lose more weight. But for the first time in my life I am really happy with my weight and myself. This is how I want to eat for the rest of my life. I feel like a new being has emerged! I never dreamed that my body would ever look and feel this healthy. I introduced my family to Natalia's program so all of us can benefit from a healthy lifestyle. Natalia, I want to thank you again for changing my life and finally helping me win the battle.

—*Elena Critean*

I've lost 20 pounds and my skin looks much younger!

—*Lesley Koustaff*

After only two weeks, I was delighted to notice I had lost 7 pounds. I also couldn't believe how much clearer and youthful looking my skin had become. My mood swings have all vanished completely.

—*Alan Stiles*

In addition to losing all my excess weight, I've noticed a tremendous improvement in my skin tone and complexion. I have more energy than when I was ten years younger and I sleep more soundly.

—*Marie Firneo*

My overall well-being has drastically improved and I feel much more energetic and stronger. I feel like my senses have awakened again. My greatest joy is that my children love to eat a fair amount of raw meals in their diet as well. When I prepare a salad with one of Natalia's delicious dressings, my three-year-old daughter always demands a large bowl for herself (and gobbles it all up). And since my children got introduced to the homemade raw ice cream they can actually pass the ice cream man on the street without tantrums.

—*Birgit Juen*

I love what Natalia has done for my daughter. I was worried about her growing into an overweight teenager and now, after working with Natalia, she is at a perfect weight for her height and age.

—*Sara Tirschwell*

I am doing great! I was between a size 14 and 12 when I started and in just three weeks I'm fitting into size 10 jeans, and according to the scale I've lost 10 pounds (and that was with clothes on!). My stomach is so much better!!

—*Jennifer Abrahmson*

I started this eating program four years ago. I lost 20 pounds and maintain the weight loss. My energy level has increased greatly and I have fewer common colds and infections.

—*W. Jacobs*

I started eating according to Natalia's principles four years ago to lose weight, improve my overall health, and expand my nutritional knowledge. Natalia helped me tremendously—I surpassed my goals. My vitality has heightened immensely and my hair and skin are noticeably more radiant.

—*S. Jacobs*

I came to Natalia's detox program overweight and unhealthy. I quickly learned a whole new way of thinking about eating which would offer me truly optimum health. Not only did I immediately lose 10 pounds (I'm still losing), but I feel so much more energetic and fulfilled. The best thing of all is that I feel like me again; feeling great about my body has made me the social being I was be-fore I put on the extra weight. There's a lot of freedom in being as beautiful as you can be, inside and out. Thank you, Natalia, for your passion, for really helping people, and for believing in me.

—*Jacqueline Vittini*

After only a month on Natalia's program, I had lost 12 pounds, my spare tire started to vanish, and my belt was buckling three holes smaller than before. Apart from the weight loss, it has been very liberating to be eating so many natural, unprocessed foods and to be more in control of what goes in my body. I have not once suffered from hunger pangs or boredom with food choices on this diet—there is always a tasty, healthful option available when you need it. Who needs processed sugar once you discover raw honey?!

—*Joe Hrbek*

THE RAW FOOD DETOX DIET. Copyright © 2005 by Natalia Rose. All rights reserved. Printed in the United States of America. No part of this book may be used or reproduced in any manner whatsoever without written permission except in the case of brief quotations embodied in critical articles and reviews. For information address HarperCollins Publishers Inc., 10 East 53rd Street, New York, NY 10022.

HarperCollins books may be purchased for educational, business, or sales promotional use. For information please write: Special Markets Department, HarperCollins Publishers Inc., 10 East 53rd Street, New York, NY 10022.

FIRST EDITION

*Designed by Kris Tobiassen*

Printed on acid-free paper

Library of Congress Cataloging-in-Publication Data has been applied for.

ISBN 0-06-079991-9

05 06 07 08 09 RRD 10 9 8 7 6 5 4

# THE RAW FOOD DETOX DIET

## THE FIVE-STEP PLAN FOR VIBRANT HEALTH AND MAXIMUM WEIGHT LOSS

### NATALIA ROSE

**Nutritionist and founder of The Raw Food Detox Diet**

ReganBooks
*An Imprint of HarperCollinsPublishers*

To my beloved husband, Lawrence,
for all the joy he brings me daily.

To God, for making the human body so
exquisite in its inherent perfection.

And also, to you, the reader, for whom I wrote this
book so you can discover your own perfection.

# ACKNOWLEDGMENTS

There are so many people who have influenced, encouraged, and loved this book into being. First and foremost, I wish to acknowledge my teacher and colleague, Gil Jacobs: my personal guide to the truth about outstanding cellular health. I also wish to acknowledge my mother who was a true health pioneer and surely influenced the path I would take to get this message out. My dear friends, Katie, Angie, and Tracey: thank you for your constant encouragement and love. To Pavia Rosati for sharing so much of her time, insight and guidance. My children, Thandi and Tommy, deserve a tremendous thanks for sharing my time and for inspiring me to adapt this program to pregnant women, and to nurture my family with natural foods. A special thanks to Christy Ferer for finding this book a home. And to Mark Sayers for the essential roll that he played. Thank you to Anna Bliss for an excellent job of editing and to Judith Regan for sharing my vision.

# CONTENTS

# FOREWORD

At first glance, the skeptic might wonder whether *The Raw Food Detox Diet* is yet another crazy fad diet. But this is really the "anti-fad" diet. Natalia Rose is bringing us back to a more natural and healthful way of eating—one for which our bodies are better suited. The overall goal of the Raw Food Detox Diet is to restore our diet to foods that are absorbed more efficiently by our digestive system.

"Diet," in the modern use of the term, has become a mantra for rapid weight loss. But studies have demonstrated that the more outlandish a diet, the more likely you are to regain any weight that you lose the moment you go off it. While Ms. Rose's program focuses on weight loss, it also emphasizes the importance of healthy, long-term results. Instead of suggesting that you dive into the most radical changes, she outlines a five-step transitional process that can apply to anyone, no matter what your current eating habits are.

The Raw Food Detox Diet provides dual health benefits for the body. First, it eliminates processed foods. Second, it promotes the intake of more fruits and vegetables. Our digestive systems do not recognize processed foods. Instead, processed foods deposit unnatural food additives in the form of toxins that are not part of our natural system. Ms. Rose's program predates the new 2005 federal government guidelines for a healthful diet, which promote significantly more fruits and vegetables, consumption of whole grains and whole foods instead of processed foods, reduced saturated fats, and lean protein sources. She actually goes further than these guidelines by suggesting how to eat in order to maximize your energy throughout the day.

As a cosmetic surgeon, my patients are always asking me how to enhance their appearance and quality of life. I can perform surgery to improve one's appearance and turn back the signs of aging with minimally invasive or surgical procedures. However, not everything can be accomplished by surgery, peels, and injections. Maintaining a healthy lifestyle is essential to maintaining a youthful look. When patients spend time, effort, and money to undergo these procedures, we try to educate them on the benefits of a healthier lifestyle to complement and even enhance the results of cosmetic surgery. In my practice, we stress the three pillars for healthy bodies: *prevention*, *treatment*, and *maintenance*. I can only offer my patients treatment and some maintenance. With a well-balanced, sensible program like The Raw Food Detox Diet, you can take preventative measures into your own hands and lead a healthier, more vibrant life.

**Dr. Steven Pearlman** *is director of the Division of Facial Plastic Surgery at St. Luke's-Roosevelt Hospital, president of the American Academy of Facial Plastic and Reconstructive Surgery, and clinical associate professor at Columbia University College of Physicians and Surgeons.*

# FOREWORD

## FRÉDÉRIC FEKKAI

I believe that natural, healthy living is the secret to inner and outer beauty. When you eat natural, raw foods, you simply look and feel better. There is no question in my mind that health maintenance must be at the core of any beauty regimen, and I recommend Natalia Rose's Raw Food Detox Diet highly. In fact, I believe in this program so much that I implemented it at my New York Salon & Spa. It is my philosophy that customers should have a comprehensive idea of beauty and health and must be well-informed so that, in addition to looking beautiful on the outside, they are healthy and happy on the inside. Simply put, healthful eating is a key component of a complete beauty regimen, not to mention a real lifestyle enhancement.

My clients who have experienced Natalia Rose's detoxification program rave about it and stick with it as a long-term lifestyle change. This is because the food is so fresh, delicious, and satisfying. I keep hearing, "Wow, this program is so great and it works!" I also really believe in getting vitamins from raw foods as opposed to taking lots of supplements. Natalia's way of nourishing the body makes intuitive sense.

As people get older, their bad habits—like smoking and eating poorly—start to show, whereas people who eat plenty of raw foods and keep their cells clean and healthy start to really stand out and look radiant despite their age. You don't have to be a vegan or eat only raw foods to do this, as Natalia will show you. It's just a matter of incorporating a few simple principles that will result in a healthier, more beautiful you.

My advice for anyone reading this book is to have fun with the whole concept of cleansing, not look at it as a chore. Sure, it takes some discipline to keep your home stocked with fresh produce, but the Raw Food Detox Diet is more than a prescription—it's a fun, fresh, and delicious way to eat and live!

*Frédéric Fekkai* *is a celebrity stylist and beauty industry pioneer. His landmark Salon & Spa, located in New York City, is one of the largest in the world. He also owns Salon & Spas in Beverly Hills and Palm Beach. Fekkai has been praised for his extensive beauty product line and is the author of* Frédéric Fekkai: A Year of Style.

## INTRODUCTION

If you are reading this book looking for the secret to a perfect body, you are going to find it. When you apply the principles in this book, you are going to uncover a thinner, younger looking, more beautiful version of your current self and experience the renewed energy of youth. You will also see a dramatic improvement in your health and a decrease in physical and mental ailments. This may sound too good to be true, but it isn't. Every single person I have worked with has radically improved his or her health and physical appearance by following the instructions contained in this book. Don't let anyone tell you it can't be done. It *can* be done. All you need is the *right* information, and you'll find that information right here.

For some of you, this book is a last resort before undertaking plastic surgery. Others may just want to lose a few pounds in preparation for a special occasion. Perhaps you are struggling with preexisting medical conditions or are overweight and under more dire pressure to reverse your health problems. This book is also for young people who have just started becoming concerned about their diet and appearance, and even those who are possibly already struggling with eating disorders. It is also for parents looking for a solution for their overweight child.

On the other hand, you may be among those readers who are not sure why they picked up this book; all you know is that you feel thick, constipated, discouraged, depressed, and in need of a little guidance and encouragement so that you can fix whatever it is that is weighing you down. For each and every one of you, this can be a haven, a place to find what you need. There is a comfortable raw food detox diet level for every unique life scenario under the sun. You may progress as slowly or as rapidly as you wish. As long as you are progressively incorporating the principles in this book, you are going to look and feel younger, healthier, leaner, and more vibrant with every passing day.

This health and weight-loss program does not require you to set a starting date or redesign your whole life. Start this very moment! You can still do anything that's on your calendar: go to restaurants, eat cooked (as opposed to all-raw) food, go to parties, take a road trip, drink wine, eat chocolate, get pregnant, anything. . . . Here's the amazing part: you do not conform to this program, *it conforms to you!* Each person that comes to me in my private practice comes with a unique life circumstance. My approach to this book will be no different. While the principles are based on the natural law that uniformly governs the physicality of us all, each person's unique state of health, lifestyle, and taste are carefully considered as this book guides you along your customized path to body heaven. But it can't start working until you make the commitment to begin.

So let's jump into that fountain of youth right now! Before a client and I start our first session together, one of the very first things I ask them do is to clear their heads of the muddy confusion of what constitutes a healthful or weight-loss-inducing food. This is not always as easy as it sounds because many dieters maintain strong attachments to their personal dietary belief system. The interesting thing about this, however, is that it is usually those very beliefs (fears about sugars, fats, calories, getting enough protein and calcium from animal products, and so forth) that created or contributed to their health and weight problems to begin with.

In this book, I am going to debunk many of these misconceptions. Soon you will see how much of what you have learned about a healthful diet is wrong. The good news is that you will soon have a better understanding of what truly contributes to rapid weight loss and vibrant health than anyone you know. After you read this book, you will have such a clear understanding of the tools for lifelong youth and beauty that you will never again get befuddled by media hype on the latest food or diet craze.

It's no surprise that almost everyone I meet complains of being utterly confused about what they should be eating when the most hyped diet concepts are not only misused but downright wrong. Take for example the concepts of soy-based foods, low-carb foods, sugars, vitamins, protein, and calcium sources. You will learn that soy-based foods are among the worst you can eat and that most of those low-carb products are the worst perpetrators of weight gain. You'll discover that raw fruit sugars can be enjoyed in large quantities and trigger excellent weight-loss results. You'll also learn that vitamin tablets are for the most part useless and that protein and calcium can be better absorbed from plant-based foods than from any animal product on the planet. It's all true and you will learn why as you read this book.

I ask my clients to "humor me" for the first hour we're together. This is when I clear their minds of this mess of information that just about everyone comes in with due to overexposure to health news information (most of which is simply PR and advertising for diet products). It's really critical that you let go of the old ideas that put you in an inferior state of health.

I am now asking you to do as I ask my private clients to do: humor me in this early stage with a "clean slate." I want you to let these grossly misunderstood diet myths drop away so that we can get to the heart of weight and aging issues. I know you will have lots of questions. Rest assured that I will, throughout the course of this book, address each and every one of these confusing issues and clarify them as they have never been wholly clarified for you before. In the meantime, it will be a challenge for us to work together if your mind is constantly triggering "pop-ups" such as "But I thought soy was supposed to be good for me?" or "But doesn't juice have a lot of sugar?" I am fully aware of what the media and popular dieting culture has fed you over the years, and none of it goes unaccounted for in these pages.

## WHY YOU ARE GOING TO LOVE THE RAW FOOD DETOX DIET

**You will never count calories, fat grams, or carb grams, or measure food again**

Conventional dieting is nothing short of sheer torture. I've been there countless times. You can't eat anything that tastes really good (not in satisfying quantities, anyway) and you're starving all the time, which means, of course, you're also grumpy all the time! The Raw Food Detox Diet is different; you are going to eat so well that you will quickly realize that you will be able to do this (with pleasure) your entire life.

**You will see results even without deliberate exercise**

While there is no doubt that our bodies need lots of motion, flexing, and fluidity for optimum performance, those of you who think you have to be a slave to an exercise regimen are in for the best news of your life: you can reach your perfect shape without any formal exercise when you apply these steps. Your skin tone will also improve because your cells are going to become healthier and tighter. Most of my Manhattan clients do a little more than the normal to-and-fro walking that the city demands.

**You will eat liberal amounts of rich, satisfying foods**

After years of eating according to this program (which followed years of mainstream dieting and the common physical ailments that go with it), I still constantly remark on how fortunate I am to have discovered this way of living and eating. My clients and I eat delicious foods in hearty, unmeasured quantities—delights that are contraband and taboo in "Dietland." Great-tasting, fulfilling eating experiences are our birthright and so is a gorgeous, healthy body. The mistake is that we think these two desirables are mutually exclusive. I'm going to show you why they need not be. But before I do, I want to give you a little sneak peek at the variety of choices you're going to enjoy when you embrace the Raw Food Detox Diet:

Avocados

Sweet potatoes

Whole grain pasta

Nuts

Dried fruits

Pure maple syrup

Fresh fruit and fresh, fruit juices

Wine

Eggs

Whole grains

Raw honey

Whole grain bread products

Raw ice cream

Raw and whole grain cookies

Raw goat cheese

Chocolate

Fish (optional)

Organic meats (optional)

Organic butter and cream

With so many online resources and exceptional new health food chain stores, you can get the items from this book's menu and recipe sections wherever you are in the world! You will also note that there is minimal preparation needed for the raw food dishes included in the recipe section. There is absolutely no need for dehydrator trays or sprouting for these decadent dishes!

### You will open the flood gates for improvements in every area of your life

I want you to think of the Raw Food Detox Diet in much larger terms than just what you eat. This program affects how you live. When you embrace the principles in this book, your life is going to improve in both large and small ways. You are going to be clearer mentally and more centered emotionally. Cleaning your body is likely going to trigger a desire to clear and cleanse your living space to reflect the inner cleansing that is taking place. You are more than likely going to feel inspired to create more clarity in your communications with others and live from a more honest space. With this inner cleansing will come a greater sense of confidence in yourself and honor for your fellow man. On a more physical level, you are going to experience greater levels of wellness and be less dependent on medications and fears relating to illness. This program is a great lifestyle enhancer in so many obvious and subtle ways—it would be impossible to name them all. Once you experience life at this level, it's unlikely that you'll want to go back to your previous habits.

**You will achieve fast results that will last—even improve—over a lifetime**

Detoxifying the body through raw foods is a way of living. The goal is not to detox and then "re-tox," but rather to learn how to love eating for constant improvement, reaching higher and higher levels of health and leanness. One of the legion problems with traditional diets is that no one wants to maintain them long term. While the Raw Food Detox Diet starts to work as early as your first meal, it's created to offer the best living experience available, so that you'll want to make this your permanent lifestyle.

## DEBUNKING TYPICAL RAW FOOD MYTHS

**Myth #1: To benefit from the raw food diet, I need to eat only raw vegan foods.**

Unlike many raw food books, *The Raw Food Detox Diet* allows and even emphasizes the inclusion of some cooked food in the diet (recommending different percentages of cooked food for each raw food transition level, as described in part II of this book). When you begin to eat raw food, it's healthy to keep some cooked food in the diet to prevent an overly intense detoxification response, to promote gastronomical pleasure and emotional satisfaction, and to take into account personal circumstance. Too often, raw food books adhere to the misguided goal of becoming a 100 percent raw foodist. In fact, that kind of diet is not for everyone, much less for those of you who are just starting out. Similarly, you will also find mention of nonvegan foods in this book. Not everyone is successful as a vegan or desires to become one. As you read, you will learn why becoming vegetarian or vegan does not guarantee health and weight-loss success.

Over the years of working with my clients, it has been clear to me that there is a place for some natural, cleanly prepared animal products within a highly raw, plant-based diet. Many of you may be committed vegans and vegetarians. You will easily adapt the detox diet to your philosophy. But for those of you who do not wish to give up every last morsel of "flesh" foods, you will learn that it is unnecessary to do so. Now that you know that you can still eat some cooked or flesh foods on this diet, you have one less excuse for not detoxing!

**Myth #2: Increasing my raw food intake means spending time soaking and sprouting nuts and dehydrating foods.**

Soaking, sprouting, and dehydration are not featured in this book and do not have to be a part of a raw foodist's routine. Why? First, moderate amounts of nuts may be enjoyed in their unsprouted state without interfering with detoxification and, as you will learn, are often easier to digest than presoaked nuts. Second, I know my audience to be a busy, hard-working, hard-playing group that wishes this process to be as easy and uncomplicated as possible. Dehydrating foods for eight or more hours is not my clients' (nor, I presume, my readers') idea of an easy long-term lifestyle regimen.

Some of you may love the idea of making your own dehydrated raw breads, cookies, and other delectable dishes, and for you there are many raw recipe books that will perfectly complement this program. But *this* book is also for those of you who wish to spend little to no time in the kitchen while you cleanse and make this way of eating a lasting lifestyle. For you it's got to be simple and delicious—no hassles! The recipes in this book were designed with these ideals at heart. You do not have to have your own raw food chef or spend more time than usual in the kitchen. Besides, demand has sparked supply. Now, many raw food companies produce exceptionally delicious, low-temperature, dehydrated raw items, or "raw treats," that anyone on a raw food diet can enjoy without going anywhere near a dehydrator tray or being forced to wait longer than it takes to undo a wrapper to get their "fix" of a mouthwatering sweet or savory raw treat.

### Myth #3: To become a raw foodist, I probably have to become a health nut—but I'm really only interested in weight loss.

*The Raw Food Detox Diet* speaks directly to weight loss. For most people, getting into raw foods is about weight loss, and this book was created to deliver the most consistent results in this area. There are tips and tricks for every level along the way so that you can avoid plateaus and get maximum results until you reach your ultimate, desired natural weight. With this diet will come a renewed sense of youth and well-being like you've never experienced before, including relief of many chronic symptoms and a dramatic increase in energy. At first, my clients are typically motivated by weight loss, but then they make the broader connection between this way of eating and feeling better than they ever have before. The Raw Food Detox Diet is, quite frankly, the most healthful diet on the planet. On the other hand, to get preachy about health and not speak to the reason most people are attracted to the raw food concept—weight loss—is not what this book is about. Your weight-loss goals are of primary focus here and you can reach them!

### Myth #4: If I just eat all raw foods, I'll be healthy and lose all my excess weight.

One of the least addressed but most critical components of successful detoxification in *The Raw Food Detox Diet* is the complete removal of the toxins that are drawn up from eating raw foods. In this book, I will guide you through simple steps that will facilitate the elimination of waste matter from your body. Contrary to popular belief, it is not what we put into our bodies that makes us healthy (various vitamins, minerals, enzymes, and so forth), but the removal of waste matter—built up from years of improper eating—that brings us into a state of glowing health. This book explains exactly how to get rid of that waste matter in the most comprehensive, efficient ways. When you do this in combination with the dietary steps, you will be able to reach a level of health and leanness that very few people in our culture ever experience.

**Myth #5: If I'm going to eat raw foods, I need to go "all raw" tomorrow.**

Finally, it is a myth that you should be able to change your lifelong eating habits overnight. *The Raw Food Detox Diet* fully appreciates the transition you are making to this way of eating and will allow you to do so very gently. For most of you this new approach to foods will be very different from what you have tried until now. I respect that it is not just your mind and desire to change that we will be working with but also your emotions, your physiology, your cravings, and your life circumstances. Taking all this into account, this book will help guide you to the perfect level of transition, leaving plenty of room for personal tastes, choices, and the speed at which you adopt the program. Absolutely anyone living on this planet can find unparalleled success on the Raw Food Detox Diet.

# HOW TO USE THIS BOOK

Start by reading part I of this book carefully in order to fully understand how your perfect body can be unveiled through the application of five simple steps. On page 61 take the test to find out your *Raw Food Transition Number*. Once you are familiar with the principles and you know your transition number, you will be presented with recommended menus for your level in part II.

Part II offers clear menu direction for all levels of readers based on their *Raw Food Transition Level*. Please note that all of the capitalized and italicized dishes mentioned throughout the book, particularly in this section, refer to recipes that appear in part III. I've provided a recipe list with page numbers on page 91 to help you locate them.

Part III offers detox recipes for every transition level, which are divided into four distinct sections: The Fundamentals are the key recipes that serve as the core for the program. They are simple but delicious, and anyone with a blender can make them. While you can still have great success on the program without them, those who incorporate them have the best results and better internal healing in the long run. The second tier of the recipe section, Expanding Your Repertoire was created especially for those of you who are more inclined toward preparing your own food and eating at home more frequently. Within this section you will find over many weight-loss-inducing, beautifying meal ideas. For the adventurous gourmand, there is a third recipe section, Masterful Creations, which is replete with still more weight-loss-inducing and beautifying recipes from my practice as a master raw foods chef. I dare you to try to run out of succulent meal ideas with this section! The fourth tier offers sample menus for entertaining.

Part IV offers detailed explanations for real-life scenarios like eating out and traveling, dealing with social situations, raising a family, and much more. Use these chapters to help you prepare for similar real-life situations.

Part V is devoted to issues that pertain specifically to aspiring raw foodists. No one who currently follows or desires to undertake a raw food diet should miss this section. As this is a lifestyle, it takes into consideration every life phase. In part V you will find easy tips for including your whole family (starting with your teens and tots) in this way of eating and living.

The appendices offer convenient resource guides for raw food products, Internet sites, stores, restaurants nationwide, and ordering information for the products mentioned throughout the book.

Finally, the approach you take to this lifestyle is very important. Some of you may be coming to this after decades of poor eating habits. Mainstream supermarket and fast-food fare are highly addictive. If unnatural substances never entered your body, you would not be out of balance and in need of tweaking today. You must take the first step in healing your body by admitting that you are addicted to these unquestionably habit-forming substances that may currently

## YOU'VE TRIED EVERY DIET OUT THERE WITH NO LONG-TERM RESULTS. WHY SHOULD THIS PROGRAM WORK IF NOTHING ELSE HAS?

Many of the clients who come to me have been chronic dieters for many years, trying anything and everything to finally tackle the weight they want to lose. The trouble with any program that does not emphasize raw foods but rather calories and fat grams is that it does not respect the natural laws of the body. The calories in/calories out approach will never cleanse the body of toxicity. So while weight may be lost in the short term and kept off with tremendous effort and restraint, the cause of a sluggish system (metabolic, digestive, circulatory, and otherwise) is never addressed. If your bodily systems are sluggish, impacted with mucosal sludge and waste matter, your organs will never function at an optimal level, and you'll always be fighting against the clock and the scale.

If, instead, you make the choice to cleanse your system of this sludge and impaction, your systems can then be liberated at the highest level, thereby increasing your ability to utilize and metabolize food. Perhaps the most important difference between this diet and traditional diets is that the latter are structured so that dieters eat concentrated starches, animal proteins, processed peanut butter, pretzels, yogurt, and pastas over a certain time period. This concentrated food only adds to the problem—it just happens to be in smaller amounts than the typical American is used to eating. Clearly, the system is going to enjoy a small break and lose weight. But without cleansing, you can never experience long-term vibrant health and a perfect body.

rule your tastes and food impulses. Simply by accepting this fact, you take the burden off your-self and realize that you are battling something bigger than mere self-control. This does not only apply to fast-food eaters. Vegans, vegetarians, and organic-consumers alike: if you are eating any refined foods, you have addictions running through your bloodstream.

You must undertake this program with an attitude of self-forgiveness. You cannot move forward in your life, much less in improving your body, until you forgive yourself for eating in such a way that has been destructive but not entirely of your own making. You must also forgive the people who have fed you unhealthful mainstream fare, as they probably didn't know any bet-ter and did the best they could at the time. Recognize that your battle with your weight has not been a fair fight up until now; you've been battling against an unseen enemy that you didn't un-derstand. But you're about to, and that will make all the difference. I trust you will enjoy your journey to the best health and body of your life.

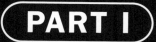

PART I

# THE RAW FOOD DETOX DIET

# DETOXIFICATION AND HOW IT WORKS

Perfect weight and a youthful appearance are the result of clean, waste-free cells—that is, cells that are free of inorganic matter. However, with our modern diet and lifestyle, clean cells are not the norm. Rather, it's much more common to find a body riddled with cells carrying matter that's not easily eliminated. This is the fundamental cause of our physical and, some would argue, mental ills. Clean, healthy cells maintain homeostasis (the healthy state of balance in the body), which keeps us feeling well. It is only when debris or waste matter from synthetic foods and overeating get lodged in our cells that our natural birthright of homeostasis turns into illness and excess weight.

Improving the caliber of your cells requires a simple process based on a simple equation. The application of even a few of the principles based on this equation will trigger your body to lose weight and feel younger as early as the very first night, with marked results in just one week. Here is the equation in its perfect simplicity:

$$Waste = Weight$$

Waste matter in the body is the fundamental source of the excess weight in your body. Get the waste out and you get the weight off. It's that easy! Imagine relieving your body of the thickness that weighs you down and makes you look prematurely old. Here's a sneak peek at how it works.

Imagine that each of your cells is a dirty room that needs cleaning. Now imagine that all of a sudden you found a team of workers that would clean those dirty rooms for you.

You wonder why you didn't look for someone to clean them before, and you hire them on the spot. After a few days, you realize those workers have already done a lot of work. The rooms that you didn't really ever believe could get clean are looking much better. But you're also wondering what you're going to do with the heaping bags of dirt and trash that have collected in the corridors of the house. You're not really going to feel the benefit of those clean rooms until that garbage is taken out. So you call up the local waste management system and ask them to come by in the morning to haul it away. They arrive on time and remove a lot of it, but they get tired and tell you that they can't take it all. They say they will try again once they've had a chance to rest and give you the number of a waste management specialist who would be more effective. You call and make an appointment for the specialist to fetch the remaining garbage (which seems the most putrid). Now you are really seeing a difference. With all the garbage out of the house, there is nothing but sunlight flooding the rooms and radiating pure joy and beauty. You can no longer tell that someone has been living there all these years. It looks like a brand new house!

Now let's fill in the analogy with the actual process of renewing your body, a.k.a. "your house." Your cells are the rooms in the house. Enzymes and organic hydration (which we will discuss at greater length) are the workers that will happily clean them. Your eliminative organs (your colon in particular), are the "local waste management" team. And finally, alternative methods of eliminating waste matter from the body (which will be described in greater detail) are the "waste management specialists."

This process of cleaning your cells is the magic formula for removing all your excess weight and restoring your body to "like new" or even "better than new" condition.

In order to start this process we need to put the workers on the payroll and get the waste management systems operating at full capacity. We can do that in five simple steps. Let's get started!

# STOP POISONING YOUR CELLS

Let's face it: we can't make any progress on yesterday's garbage if we are constantly cleaning up after today's mess. To make any difference at all, you simply need to bring less garbage into your body today than you did yesterday. To make a significant difference, you need to eliminate as much of the garbage from your diet as you possibly can. What is garbage? It is anything that your body cannot fully utilize and/or eliminate. Garbage is anything that will get stored in your body because it is not coming out. It is like Styrofoam in a landfill. Garbage goes by many names, including "waste," "toxins," and "debris." I will use these terms interchangeably.

After my initial discussions with new clients, one of the first things I do is take them to a high-quality grocer—one that is stocked with some organic produce and a range of natural foods—like Whole Foods (see appendix for help finding a health food store near you) and show them how easy it is to find items that work as excellent substitutions for their favorite mainstream food tastes, flavors, and textures. I call these items "transition foods." Transition foods can be both raw and nonraw foods that give you all the satisfaction you are looking for in your diet without inhibiting (and therefore actually aiding) detoxification.

Below is a list of the transition foods and corresponding brands that I recommend. Their primary role is to take the place of the foods you eliminate from your diet at this initial stage, as you learn to stop poisoning your cells so that cleansing can begin to take place. For many of you, these transition foods will be your staple foods for decades to come. Some of them are of a higher caliber than others, so your list may become more nuanced as you progress. Whatever level you reach, there will always be room in your diet for these high-quality transition foods, that is, foods with minimal processing. The best thing about them is that they are emotionally as well as physically satisfying. Many of them act as comfort foods that enable the program to work easily for everyone.

# RAW FOOD DETOX DIET TRANSITION FOODS

| TRANSITION FOOD | RECOMMENDED BRAND |
|---|---|
| Sprouted grain breads | Alverado St. Bakery or Ezekiel* |
|     Sprouted grain bagels | |
|     Sprouted grain tortillas | |
|     Sprouted grain pitas | |
| Chips | Guiltless Gourmet* |
| Chocolate chip cookies | Joseph's* |
| Carob chip cookies | Kollar Cookies |
| Oatmeal raisin cookies | Kollar Cookies |
| Crackers | Ak-Mak * |
| Sweet raw treats | (see appendix for list) |
| Granola | Lydia's Raw Granola** |
| Raw granola bars | Blessing's Raw Granola bars** |
| Spicy-salty raw flax seed crackers | Blessing's or Glaser Farms |
| Whole grain pasta | Eden Foods* |
| Soba noodles | any brand |
| Pasta sauce | Seeds of Change* |
| Organic vegetable broth (use to cook with in place of butter or oil) | Pacific* |
| Raw almond butter | Bazini* |
| Raw tahini | Marantha's* |
| Sprouted Grain Dense Cake Bread | Manna: Multi-Grain* |

Almond milk ...............................................Pacific*

Organic unsalted butter...........................Horizons*

Goat milk ice cream................................Red Acre Farms

Goat cheese............................................Alta Dena*

Soy sauce ...............................................Nama Shoyu*

Apple cider vinegar ................................Tree of Life*

Apple juice concentrate ..........................Bernard Jensen's

Cold-pressed olive oil .............................Biorganic or Spectrum*

Stone-pressed olive oil ...........................Bariani

Sweet potatoes ......................................Any brand

Brown rice..............................................Any brand

Legumes and legume-based soups ..........Taste Adventure*

All whole grains:
>     Millet
>     Quinoa
>     Barley
>     Wheat berries

Fresh fish (ideally wild or organic)

Organic chicken

High-quality meats (i.e., the best cuts and organic filet mignon over ground beef.)

Raw nuts or seeds

Sulfur-free dried fruit

> *Should be stocked at most Whole Foods Markets and other health food stores nationwide.
> **Stocked at High Vibe Health & Healing (www.highvibe.com/raw).
> (See the appendix for more information on where to find delicious, satiating raw food products!)

Here are some important tips to help you maximize your efforts when you are transitioning to these higher quality, nontoxic foods.

# RAW FOOD DETOX SHOPPING TIP SHEET

1. Make several copies of the transitional foods list for your purse, car, fridge, and office.

2. If the nearest health food store is a long distance away, save the wrappers of the transitional food items you like. You can either ask your local market to order and carry them or call the companies directly for bulk shipments (which are typically much cheaper at wholesale).

3. Look for farming cooperatives, which offer a vast assortment of fresh fruits and vegetables at great prices.

4. Shop from your impulses in the produce aisle, not from habit. Don't just buy apples because you always buy apples. When just the thought of a fresh pineapple gets you salivating, buy one. Plan to buy at least one new fruit and vegetable every week. (This is a great way to get kids to eat fresh fruits and vegetables, too. Let them choose the item and find a recipe for it!)

5. Don't focus on what you can't have. Focus on everything you *can* have!

6. Clean out your kitchen cabinets of all the junk you will be eliminating before filling them with your raw transition foods. You can leave one cupboard and one shelf in the fridge for items that your family members may not be ready to part with. Don't threaten them with the loss of their kitchen real estate! (For more on detoxifying your kitchen, see page 191.)

7. Get to know the produce and bakery managers at your grocery store. The produce managers will be able to help you find the freshest items and even order items they don't currently carry. The bakery managers are usually in charge of ordering the category of foods that I call "raw treats," the raw gourmet packaged items that are so helpful to this lifestyle.

8. Seek out the nearest health food store. Health food stores are *not* the GNCs and vitamin stores of the world. I'm talking about those seventies-style, granola, "smells like vitamin $B_{12}$" shops across the country. These stores will have almost everything on the transition foods shopping list

and will be most likely to carry the raw food items you want. Every city in America has at least one, but often you might miss it if you're not looking for it.

**9.** Buy more produce than you think you will need. Once you start trying the raw dressings and sauces in the upcoming recipe section, you will want seconds and thirds of your salads. You'll be eating a lot of fruit, too. A hearty appetite is a good sign in this diet, so be sure you have enough fresh food on hand to satisfy it.

**10.** Take new pleasure in the shopping process. We all live hectic lives, but try not to look at shopping for your food as a hassle. Allow your spirit to guide you to positive new food choices that truly delight you. Breathe deeply if you're forced to wait in long lines. Imagine where the fruits and

---

### HIGH-PROTEIN DIET BARS AND SHAKES
### WILL PACK ON POUNDS AND INVITE DISEASE

I find it mind-boggling that diet and health enthusiasts of today reach for Myoplex bars, Keto-chips, and soy protein shakes in an effort to attain a lean, powerful physique. Ask an average American to choose which is the better food choice, a Power Bar or an avocado, and he/she will likely point out that the Power Bar has 200 calories and 2 grams of fat while the avocado has 400 calories and 14 grams of fat, and therefore choose the Power Bar.

But the body regards these two items very differently. To the Power Bar, it says, "That's sugar and chemicals, which I can't break down. That will cause me to store waste and gain weight." But to the avocado it says, "Oh, I know exactly what to do with you. I can break you down completely!" So you see, the number of calories, protein grams, fat grams, and carb grams are not the information you need to make informed choices about what to put in your body.

You've been told for decades to read nutrition labels, but you probably haven't been reading the right part of the label. Forget the counts and read the ingredients. Or, better yet, when you think of putting something into your mouth, ask yourself, "Is this food in its natural state and is its source recognizable?" If the answer is "no," put it down. If the answer is "yes," go to town!

vegetables came from, how you will prepare them, how they will taste, and finally how they will help you to detox your body and achieve physical perfection!

The following old-school "diet" foods are guaranteed to *squash* weight-loss attempts and cause premature aging/cellular degeneration:

- All fat-free yogurts (frozen and otherwise)

- Sugar-free flavored yogurt (all varieties, but particularly the leading brands)

- Weight-loss bars (including Luna, Power Bars, Zone, Keto, etc.)

- Packaged, processed cold cuts

- Frozen waffles

- All manufactured low-carb weight-loss items

- Crystal Light

- All diet sodas

- Milk (including skim)

- All frozen lean-style dinners

- Sugar-free Jell-O and frozen desserts

- Sugar-free hot cocoa

- "Light" white bread

Regardless of how low the carbohydrate or calorie count, the above foods cannot be fully digested by the body, so they will get stored as *waste*. As you now know, Waste = Weight! Besides, you could be eating real food with truly satisfying textures and tastes like avocados, sweet potatoes, real full-fat cream and butter, dates, macadamia nuts, and much more while actually losing waste/weight and feeling like you're twelve years old again. Try achieving *that* with constipating mainstream diet food!

"But we encounter poisons in the environment every day," you may be thinking. That's true, but on a largely raw, natural diet, our body can deal more effectively with those toxic elements. If you ingest processed foods and fats on top of a largely cooked food diet (vegetarian included), you're subjecting yourself to a double whammy that your body will find very difficult to handle.

I know it's tempting to think that eating foods labeled "nonfat" will make you lean, but I hope that you will never fall into that trap again. What you want to look for when buying pre-pared foods are the ingredients, *not* the number of fat grams or calories. Remember that natural foods are recognizable by the body and can be broken down, whereas unnatural substances can-not be broken down and will actually contribute to the slowing of your metabolism, degenera-tion of your organs, weight gain, and premature aging.

This simple point is extremely empowering. It means you'll never again have to look at anything other than the ingredients in a product to know whether or not it is good for your body. If it has refined flour, sugar, heated oils (any oils that are not specifically labeled "cold-pressed" or "stone-pressed") or chemicals in it, it is not fit for human consumption.

See the hierarchy of foods that I've listed below. Commit this to memory and evaluate the food you eat accordingly. This hierarchy is based on the very simple philosophy that the most healthful foods for the body are the easiest foods to digest. I like to call them "quick exit foods"—foods that pass through the body, leaving the least amount of residue that can be turned into waste matter. You will see that hydrating fresh fruits and vegetables are at the top of the list.

# QUICK EXIT HIERARCHY OF FOOD
### (1 = best, 11 = worst)

1. Raw fruits and vegetables (preferably organic) such as apples, grapes, melons, bananas, avocados, romaine lettuce, cucumbers, carrots, kale, tomatoes, etc.; raw honey, stevia (a natural sweetener)

2. Lightly-steamed, low-starch vegetables (all vegetables other than white potatoes, acorn and butternut squash, and pumpkin); pure maple syrup, agave nectar
   *Note that corn and legumes are starches, not vegetables.*

3. Organic raw nuts and seeds (almonds, pine nuts, walnuts, macadamia nuts, sesame seeds, sunflower seeds, etc.)

4. Raw stone-pressed or cold-pressed plant oils (especially olive oil, though hemp seed and flax seed oils are also acceptable)

5. Cooked starchy vegetables (sweet potatoes, butternut and acorn squash, pumpkin, etc.)

6. Raw unpasteurized dairy products (particularly from goats and sheep)

7. Whole grains (brown rice, millet, whole wheat, buckwheat, etc.)

8. Pasteurized dairy and animal flesh (preferably limited to organic fish and minimal organic meat and poultry products)

9. All non-whole grain flour products (white bread, white rice, white pasta, white pizza dough, flour tortillas, etc.); sugar (white sugar, brown sugar, corn syrup, etc.)

10. Cooked animal fats/hydrogenated oils (lard, cooked oils, etc.), mainstream meats, poultry; soy products

11. Chemicals, artificial coloring and sweeteners (aspartame, saccharine, unnatural additives of all kinds)

Eating within Quick Exit Food levels 1 to 8 is acceptable in the Raw Food Detox Diet program and doable for anyone. You will reach the highest levels of health when you eat within levels 1 to 5, but you can work your way up to those levels (if that is your goal) at your own pace.

## THE BIG FAT TRUTH

There is much confusion about what makes a "good" fat. It's actually really simple. A good fat is a *raw* fat, whereas all other fats are damaging. You no longer need to know the difference between a saturated fat, a monounsaturated fat, or a partially hydrogenated fat. All you need to know is whether it's a cooked or unheated fat. Here is a list of good raw fat sources:

- Cold-pressed oils

- Raw avocado

- Raw nuts

- Raw coconut and coconut butter

While not raw, you may also use organic butter and cream in small quantities. Despite fat's bad reputation, it is one of the essential components of optimum health and longevity. Raw plant

## SOY IS THE MOST MUCUS-FORMING PLANT FOOD ON THE PLANET!

Soy has received a huge amount of press over the last decade. It has been touted as nothing short of a miracle food. Before you slurp back a glass of soy milk in lieu of another mainstream beverage, consider this: soy is the most mucus-forming plant food on the planet. The form of mucus it creates is called mucoid matter—not to be confused with mucus membrane. This mucus is a sticky, sludge-like substance that holds up the body's flow and productivity. It accumulates and creates respiratory distress in asthmatics, creates common digestive problems like IBS (irritable bowel syndrome), and, by slowing down the body's digestion and circulation systems, ultimately triggers weight gain and premature aging.

You are probably wondering about all those healthy Japanese, who are supposedly living on soy. The truth is, the Japanese do not eat nearly as much soy as soy product manufacturers would have you believe. More to the point, they do not eat the same heavily processed soy products that Americans eat, like imitation chicken and pseudo-fish. They are eating edamame pods (soy in its natural, unprocessed state) and small amounts of tofu. Americans misinterpret this to mean that every product listing soy as an ingredient is automatically a "free, guiltless food" with myriad magical properties. It's a wonder we don't walk on water after consuming them! Soy sauce is fine because it isn't concentrated, meaning it is a liquid rather than a dense food. You may also employ small amounts of raw miso in recipes. But other than that, you will want to avoid all processed soy products, unless you want to keep reaching for that inhaler!

fats, greens, and sweet fruits are the three building blocks of optimum health. In order for you to be naturally lean and clean, you need raw plant fats in your diet. I know some of you have been avoiding fat for as long as you can remember, and it's really difficult to free yourself from your preconceptions. But once you see how well all of these detoxifying principles work, you'll begin to expand your diet to include these precious fats.

It's really unfortunate that we have been conditioned to avoid some of the most valuable foods available to us in nature, such as avocados and raw nuts, for fear of their fat content. I encourage you to evaluate food on its tendency to leave waste residue in the body. If it is a natural food, consumed in its natural, raw, and properly combined state, it will not leave waste residue. Inversely, if the food is unnatural and ill-combined, it will be more likely to leave waste behind.

# WHAT ABOUT DAIRY?

Now, don't have a cow but . . . the milk you think is so good for you and your bones is actually contributing to the deterioration of your bones, organs, and waistline—yes, even skim milk! Regular cow's milk products are the biggest culprits and should be avoided at all costs. But goat and sheep dairy products are acceptable, particularly if they are raw. For example, there is an excellent cheddar-style raw goat cheese made by a California dairy called Alta Dena. This cheese is stocked in most health food stores nationwide. It is delicious and fully satisfying for all you cheese lovers out there!

There are two things that make cow's milk products so bad. First, the protein molecule in cow's milk is too difficult for the human body to break down, which means it will leave waste residue in the body and really pile up if you consume it regularly. Remember, cow's milk was designed for baby cows—not humans! Second, the milk is pasteurized, so any good attributes it may have had are cooked out, including its enzymes.

A bit of good news, however, is that butter and cream—since they do not contain the casein-heavy protein—are much easier to break down and are acceptable in small quantities. Nut milks, like almond or hazelnut, will quickly replace your need for cow milk. If you're up for it, you can even make your own nut milk (blend 1 part nuts with 3 parts water, and strain through a cheesecloth) or you can buy the Pacific brand nut milks, which are delicious and store very well. In terms of your calcium needs, consider this:

- In order for calcium to be properly absorbed and not leached from the bones, magnesium is needed. Dairy products contain very little magnesium. Leafy greens contain calcium and magnesium in perfect ratio for optimal calcium absorption.

- Despite the fact that American women have been consuming an average of two pounds of milk per day for their entire lives, according to the National Institute of Disability and Research, it is estimated that 30 percent of postmenopausal white women in the United States have osteoporosis of the spine, hip, or arm![1]

- According to the European Vegetarian Union, "Vegetarian women were also shown to have a much lower risk for and a lesser degree of postmenopausal osteoporosis. The Chinese vegetarian women tested only consume about one-third the amount of calcium European women do, but in their case, all the calcium is derived from plant foods instead of dairy products, as is often the case in western countries. Osteoporosis as we know it is virtually unknown in this area and not one of the women tested had this disease!"[2]

■ According to Australia's *Nexus Magazine* (November 1998), "The Bantu of Africa have the lowest rates of osteoporosis of any culture, yet they consume from 175 to 476 mg of calcium daily. The Japanese average about 540 mg daily, but the early post-menopausal spinal fractures so common in the West are almost unheard of in Japan. Overall, their spinal fracture rate is one-half that of the United States. All this is true, even though the Japanese have one of the longest life spans of any population. Studies of populations in China, Gambia, Ceylon, Surinam, Peru, and other cultures all report similar findings of low calcium intake and low osteoporosis rates. Anthropologist Stanley Garn, who studied bone loss over a fifty-year period in people in North and Central America, failed to find a link between calcium intake and bone loss."[3]

■ The growth hormones and antibiotics that are injected into cows to produce milk enter directly into our bloodstream when we consume milk products. Even most organic dairies use these hormones—just in smaller amounts.

■ Milk is one of the most mucus-forming foods we can consume. Knowing this, it should come as no surprise that American children suffer to such a great extent from asthma, allergies, ear infections, and colds. Reared on formula, cow's milk, and dairy-rich diets, their bodies become laden with mucus buildup in just a few short years. World-renowned physician and best-selling author Dr. Christine Northrup states, "Dairy is a tremendous mucus producer and a burden on the respiratory, digestive, and immune systems." She says when patients "eliminate dairy products for an extended period and eat a balanced diet, they suffer less from colds and sinus infections."[4]

■ According to Victorias Kulvinskas, cofounder of the Hippocrates Institute and best-selling author, pasteurized diary and cooked meat cause our white blood cell count to increase by 300 to 400 percent. This is what happens when the body responds to infection![5]

■ Dairy can block iron absorption resulting in a reduced red-blood cell count, which causes anemia.

■ Pasteurized dairy intake is linked to thyroid conditions and diabetes.

■ While dairy products do contain calcium, they also contain difficult-to-digest animal proteins, lactose sugar, growth hormones, and numerous other contaminants.

Since eliminating dairy from your diet can be a very big step, many of you will continue to consume it. At the very least, you can learn how to combine it properly with other foods. Dairy combines best with raw and cooked vegetables. Therefore, if you would like to enjoy cheese as part of your meal, make a big raw salad topped with your favorite natural cheese. Goat cheese and goat milk are superior to cow-based dairy products, as the protein in goat milk is much easier for humans to digest. Goat milk is often used as a more natural substitute to mother's milk for infants and toddlers. Raw goat- and cow-milk cheeses are always preferable to regular pasteurized cheese.

The most healthful sources of calcium are leafy, green vegetables like kale, dandelion, and Swiss chard, which are high in *absorbable* calcium, not to mention a host of other healthful nutrients. Drink your Green Lemonade (see page 48) every day and you'll never have to worry about the health of your bones.

## WHAT ABOUT VITAMINS?

It seems that every day a new study is released indicating the effectiveness of one vitamin or another. This sends consumers into a mad frenzy of purchasing what they are led to believe is the wonder element that will prevent aging, improve brain function, prevent disease, and generally work miracles.

The good news is that, if you are eating a diet high in raw plant foods and juice greens on a daily basis, you are getting all of nature's essential elements and do not need to concern yourself with what I call "nutri-hype trend stories." According to a press release of September 21, 2004,

### A WORD ABOUT ALCOHOL AND COFFEE

I definitely recommend avoiding hard liquor as it interferes with detoxification by being too harsh on the liver. On the other hand, while coffee is definitely highly acid-forming, it will not interfere with your detoxification in the first year. I recommend giving it up, but liquids like coffee and wine are not your biggest battle. It's the damaging "concentrated" foods like white flour, large amounts of animal flesh, and packaged foods—foods that leave undigested waste in the body—that pose the biggest threat to your health and hinder weight loss.

by the Subcommittee on Human Rights and Wellness, a report sponsored by the FDA estimates that "American consumers spend $80 billion annually on dietary supplements, and there are about 29,000 products on the market—with another thousand new products introduced each year"[6] (www.house.gov/reform). The health and diet industry takes full advantage of the fact that the general public is highly ignorant about nutrition by convincing them that they need the latest "super nutrients" pill.

Supplements are just that: supplemental nutrition for bodies that are not getting adequate nutrition from their daily dietary intake. If you're eating of nature's bounty every day, you don't need to supplement your diet with pills. In fact, people who think that they can eat the standard American diet and then get away with popping a few vitamins are in for a very unpleasant surprise because doing this does not ensure their nutritional needs are met.

Vegetable juice is the best vitamin and mineral source available. Drink it often and you will not have to worry about getting enough of the right nutrients. More important, when your cells are clean, they are going to absorb nutrients much better. Everything falls into place and hypes are put to rest when you eat according to nature's plan.

# EAT QUICK EXIT FOODS IN QUICK EXIT COMBINATIONS

Now that you have stopped poisoning your cells, it's time for you to learn the secret to eating for weight loss and constant waste elimination. At the core of this secret is your digestive system. If your digestive system is able to move food through very quickly (thus eliminating it quickly), you will minimize the waste matter that can accumulate in your body and avoid weight gain for the rest of your life!

The first thing you want to do is eat foods that are the easiest to digest and move out of the body. (Please refer to the Quick Exit Hierarchy of Food on page 27.) The second thing to do is eat these foods in "quick exit combinations." This means that when you make a meal out of high-quality, quick exit foods, the combinations of the foods in your meal should also be as easy as possible to digest. As you've learned, the quicker the food is digested, the less waste matter it will leave. But it's equally important to remember that if you're eating foods that take a long time to be digested, your body's energy and resources are being wasted on breaking down meals rather than helping your body to renew and cleanse.

In addition to helping you lose weight, eating in quick exit combinations can relieve digestive problems such as acid reflux, gassiness, constipation, IBS, and more. Once you learn to eat in quick exit combinations, you will immediately begin to feel energized and the pounds will begin to drop off!

## SLOW VERSUS QUICK EXIT COMBINATION TRANSIT TIMES

Certain foods, when eaten together, take two to three times as long to digest as other food combinations. For example, an avocado on a piece of toast (a good quick exit combination) requires only three to four hours in the stomach, whereas that same piece of toast combined with an egg requires upward of eight hours in the stomach—and that's just the stomach, not the entire digestive tract (clearly, a slow exit combination). After enjoying a quick exit combination, your body can quickly get back to work strengthening and rejuvenating itself, whereas a slow exit combination will draw all your energy to your stomach for hours on end and leave you feeling less vibrant.

What happens over a lifetime of mixing slow exit foods in slow exit combinations? Think of eight-hour food combinations being ingested three times a day. A major backlog develops, turning a healthy, clean digestive tract and healthy cells into a veritable cesspool where bacteria can thrive and the whole of the eliminative channels (liver, skin, kidneys, colon, spleen) slows down. As you may have guessed, this leads straight to constipation, acne, asthma, arthritis, and more. Poor digestion and the excess waste matter that is connected to it is at the root of everything from minor complaints such as heartburn and gas to more serious physical issues like thyroid disorders and circulation problems. And since these ailments are creating a further drain on your body's energy supply, you are being robbed of your youthfulness and beauty with every ill-combined meal you eat.

## QUICK EXIT COMBINATIONS

There are four basic categories of foods for our purposes: (1) starches, (2) fleshes, (3) nuts/seeds/dried fruit, and (4) fresh fruit. Eating in quick exit combinations means that with very few exception these four categories of foods should not mix with one another in the stomach (in the same meal or in too short a time period before or after a meal). Therefore starches should not mix with fleshes; fleshes should not mix with nuts/seeds/dried fruits; and likewise, nuts/seeds/dried fruits should never come in contact with starches. The first three categories may be mixed with unlimited amounts of raw vegetables. The first two categories may be mixed with cooked vegetables as well. Fresh fruit can be mixed with raw vegetables but, for best results, should really not mix with anything else. Ideally, these four groups should never touch one another in the stomach.

# QUICK EXIT COMBINATION TABLE

(Never mix these four categories with one another with a few exceptions.)

| STARCHES | FLESHES (FLESH-PROTEIN) | NUTS/SEEDS/ DRIED FRUITS (FAT-PROTEIN) | FRESH FRUITS |
|---|---|---|---|
| Whole grain breads | Fish | Raw nuts | Citrus |
| Brown rice | Eggs | Raw seeds | Bananas (combine well with fresh as well as dried fruits) |
| Sweet potatoes | Chicken | Raw, unsulfured dried fruits (combine well with raw nuts/seeds but should otherwise only be enjoyed alone or with raw vegetables, always on an empty stomach) | |
| Avocados (technically a fruit but combines with starches and dried fruits) | Meat (beef, lamb, pork, etc.) | | Plums |
| | Game | | Nectarines |
| | Shellfish | | Grapes |
| Legumes (lentils, cooked peas, beans, etc.) | Raw cheese (while it should ideally only be combined with vegetables, some people can get away with combining it with flesh) | | Berries |
| Cooked corn (raw corn combines as a vegetable) | | Mature coconut (small and brown) | Other fruits |
| Young coconut (large and green, or shaved; also combines with raw nuts/dried fruits) | | | |
| Pasta | | | |

Keep in mind that each person's digestive system is unique. The best way to tell if a food combines well for you is to experiment on yourself. If your stomach is calm and gas-free after a given combination and you continue to lose weight, then that combination is okay for you.

If you want to get more serious about this, there are stricter rules for quick exit combinations. For example, ideally one would not eat cheese and flesh together, or tomatoes with grains, or bananas with cantaloupe. However, it is important to realize that your body is probably not yet clean enough to notice these far subtler nuances in food combinations. For most people, it can take years before these rules will apply. What I've laid out in the above table will work, giving you room for pleasure without sacrificing results. These four food groups are the "biggies" and if you get this much right, you will transform your body!

## QUICK EXIT COMBINATION TIPS

1. Foods in different categories should never be mixed in the same meal, but foods in the same category may be enjoyed at the same meal.

2. Avocados are also unique in that they are technically a fruit but combine as a starch. They can also combine with dried fruits but not with nuts. This is an interesting exception that should be well noted.

3. Fruit should only be consumed on an empty stomach—at least 3 hours after a properly combined meal (or ideally, as your morning meal). Your new fruit mantra: "Eat it alone or leave it alone."

4. Fresh fruit only takes twenty to thirty minutes to exit the stomach completely, so you may enjoy another category of food thirty minutes after consuming fresh fruit.

5. Bananas are special in that they cross over several categories. They combine well with both fresh fruit and dried fruit as well as with avocados. Note that bananas require approximately forty-five minutes in the stomach as opposed to thirty minutes for other fresh fruit.

6. Never eat fresh fruit for dessert after a cooked meal as it will cause fermentation.

7. Wait three to four hours after eating before switching food groups.

8. If you have a very large appetite, eat more within the same food type. For example, you're better off having two pieces of fish or two plates of whole grain pasta with vegetables instead of introducing a different food category—or eating three sweet potatoes instead of one sweet potato with a piece of fish, chicken, or other flesh.

9. All vegetables (except high-starch vegetables such as sweet potatoes, acorn, or butternut squash) may be enjoyed with flesh dishes.

10. All vegetables may be enjoyed with starch meals.

11. Nuts, seeds, and dried fruits go better with raw vegetables than cooked vegetables.

12. Dairy can be combined with flesh in most cases.

13. Nut butters should not be placed on grain breads.

14. When eating an exclusively raw meal, beginners can get away with mixing starches (like avocados) and raw nuts or preparing recipes with small amounts of fresh fruit (like the Apple-Raisin Dream and Arame Salad—see recipe section) because there are plenty of enzymes to help digestion.

15. Raw corn combines as a vegetable; cooked corn combines as a starch. You can eat unlimited amounts of raw corn—enjoy it right off the cob in the summertime!

16. If you are going to "miscombine" a meal, do it at dinner so your body has plenty of time to move it through the stomach before the next meal comes through.

17. Starch meals should only include the highest-quality starches (whole grains, sprouted grain breads, sweet potatoes, and so forth).

18. Don't let the hard-core rules of eating mono-meals and keeping different fruit categories separate discourage you. These rules are not important at this stage. Focus on enjoying your meals and improving your food choices.

19. Dagoba and Green & Black's 70-percent chocolate bars make the perfect dessert for any food category. (These products are 70-percent pure chocolate, meaning they contain less sugar, milk, or other ingredients that make chocolate a "no-no" at a lower percentage.)

20. Condiments, 70-percent chocolate, nut milks, and of course all raw vegetables are neutral, which means they can be mixed with any food category except fruit.

## Slow Exit Combination

Here's what happens when you mix foods from different categories. Whenever you eat a flesh food, the stomach sends up the acidic flesh/protein digesting enzyme pepsin, which initiates protein digestion. When you eat a starch food (a concentrated carbohydrate), the stomach sends out an alkaline medium to digest it. The acid and alkaline substances neutralize each other so digestion is severely hindered, causing fermentation.

What happens to this backlog of poorly digested meals in your body? When proper digestion cannot take place, the food in the digestive system putrefies and ferments. This is not simply from one day of poor combinations but a lifetime of improper eating. Bacteria thrive on putrefactive matter and the whole of the eliminative channels slows down, leading to constipation and/or diarrhea, two ailments that millions of Americans suffer from daily.

If the body's energy is being wasted on digestion, then it cannot be as effective at fighting illness, building immunity, and maintaining general upkeep of cells, tissues, and organs. Again, this is a critical point in terms of weight loss because this backlog of waste from miscombined meals holds up the elimination process. This putrefactive waste matter is the dieter's worst enemy because where elimination is poor, weight loss is slow and weight gain, sluggishness, and poor circulation are inevitable.

You're probably wondering what you're going to be able to eat now that many typical food combinations have been eliminated. You will have more to eat that you can imagine! And best of all, when you're properly combining, you don't have to worry about amounts—you can finally eat to satisfaction! You can enjoy most of your favorite foods, just not all of them at the same time. For example, if you would like pasta for dinner (a starch), you may enjoy whole grain pasta with marinara sauce and unlimited vegetables. Feel free to order side portions of vegetables like steamed broccoli, carrots, spinach, and/or a raw salad to ensure you feel satisfied. Again, hardcore raw food theorists would argue that tomatoes (acidic) would interfere with starch (alkaline) digestion, but this is not an issue for most people. If you find it makes you gassy, then don't do it. (Gassiness is a good way to gauge whether something is a bad combination.) If you are going to your favorite seafood restaurant, you may enjoy your favorite fish with plenty of vegetables and salad, but you should not eat it with a starch or carbohydrate such as rice, bread, potatoes, grains, couscous, and so forth.

Don't worry, it's really easy once you get the hang of it! Don't let this concept of food combining intimidate you or prevent you from trying it. It is the single most effective principle for effortless weight loss and, if you give it a week, you will see how easy it can be. Don't worry if you mess up. You don't have to be perfect. I do recommend that if you plan on miscombining now and then, do so at dinner. Miscombining at lunch will likely sap your energy for the rest of the day since you probably won't wait eight hours before your evening meal, and you will only add to the problem by putting a full meal on top of a fermented lunch. If you miscombine in the evening, your digestive system will have the whole night to deal with it. In this case, it's always a good idea to wait until you've moved your bowels in the morning before taking in anything new.

An easy way to think about leaving enough time between different food groups is to imagine that you want each meal to have fully departed the stomach before the next meal is sent in. If your meals—consisting of the highest-quality foods—exit your body with space between them (no pile-ups), then you cannot put on extra weight. However, you can put on weight or impede weight loss by improperly combining the best quality foods or properly combining the worst quality foods. Your digestive system works much like a highway; you want to avoid a traffic jam.

## A Word about Beans

Nature combines both starch and protein in beans and legumes, which means that while they are a natural plant food, they are not easy to digest. For weight loss or for anyone with bowel issues, I recommend avoiding starchy legumes (but note that raw snow peas and green beans are vegetables). If you enjoy beans, keep in mind that they are more starch than protein and combine better with vegetables and other starches than with protein. So, for example, if you are a fan of Mexican food or find yourself stuck in a Mexican or Tex-Mex restaurant, a tostada with lots of greens, salsa, and beans would be an excellent choice. Feel free to top it off with some guacamole, but avoid the sour cream and cheese.

## Neutral Foods

Neutral foods can be mixed with anything except fresh fruit. All raw vegetables are neutral, as is 70-percent chocolate. Condiments like mustard and soy sauce are neutral as are olives, olive oil, and all herbs, spices, and other seasonings. Almond milk and other nut milks are also neutral, as is hot chocolate made with nut milk. Raw honey and pure maple syrup are neutral (although many hard-core raw foodists advocate eating honey only on its own, it is not a problem for me or my clients). Lemons and tomatoes are not technically neutral as they can acidify alkaline foods, but I use them as neutral foods without a problem.

## Why Fresh Fruit Does Not Mix with Any Other Food

Most fruit requires twenty to thirty minutes to pass through the stomach (melons take slightly less time, bananas slightly more). If eaten with another food type, such as cottage cheese, fresh fruit is held back because the cottage cheese needs at least three and up to four hours in the stomach to digest. The fruit will ferment with the cheese causing much trouble.

**A HEALTHFUL FOOD IS DETERMINED NOT BY HOW MANY VITAMINS IT HAS, BUT BY HOW QUICKLY AND THOROUGHLY IT CAN LEAVE THE BODY.**

One of the first things my clients learn when they work with me is how easy it is to determine a healthful food. They no longer have to look to the five o'clock news to find out the latest trend food for health and weight loss. They know more from one simple fact than from 100 diet broadcasts: a truly healthful food is a food that makes a quick exit out of the body. This is a bit of a revelation for most people because they've been led to believe that a healthful food "sticks to your ribs" or "really stays with you all morning," as in the case of oatmeal. Hear this: a food that the body can take in, assimilate, and then quickly discard—a quick exit food—is a monumentally healthful food. This means that foods like watermelon and leafy greens are the most healthful foods on the planet. So why are we eating so much soy and chicken? As a culture, we say that we know that fruits and vegetables are the most healthful foods, yet how many of us really apply that knowledge?

### The Fat-Protein Category

Fat-proteins are nuts and seeds. Ideally, they should be kept separate from animal protein and starches. If that's too difficult for you at this early stage, just treat nuts and seeds like a regular protein and keep them separate from starches at the very least. Like starches and proteins, fat-proteins may be enjoyed with all kinds of nonstarchy vegetables. They also combine well with *dried* fruit (but not with fresh fruit). Nuts and seeds have long been considered a protein food, but they are actually predominantly fat. This is not a reason to avoid them! Raw nuts and seeds can actually mobilize bad fats, encourage elimination of free radicals, and correct thyroid imbalances, thereby contributing to weight loss! (Free radicals damage healthy cells, leading to cancer and premature aging.)

# QUICK EXIT DESSERTS

I love the way my clients' faces light up when I tell them about all the sweet things they will be able to enjoy as they embark on the program. I love being the bearer of the news that they can

## PEANUTS AND SOY NUTS

Peanuts and soy nuts are not part of the approved nut category. They are simply too difficult to digest in addition to being addictive and mucus-forming. Due to their high-protein content and low cost, they have gained a coveted place as America's "national health food." (I don't even want to think about what the "national junk food" is!) Peanuts are not a health food. In fact, they are not even nuts. Peanuts are legumes. Like soy nuts, peanuts should be avoided at all costs.

enjoy 100-percent pure maple syrup, thick raw honey, stevia, agave nectar, and dates as sweetening agents with little concern for quantity. Almost every one yearns for the sweetness in nature, but so many of you have been desperately calorie- and carb-counting for such a long time that you have been terribly deprived of this pleasure. I know the relief you are going to feel knowing that you can enjoy sweet things again—and not by using some carcinogenic saccharin-laden packet that is falsely luring you into a sense of "sweet" security while it piles indigestible toxicity into your cells! The sweets in the Raw Food Detox Diet are safe, natural, and delicious. They are the best of all worlds.

Here's how you can properly combine your delicious desserts guilt-free. When eating a starch-based meal, you can enjoy a high-quality spelt or other grain cookie sweetened with pure maple syrup, like the Kollar Cookie brand (*www.kollarcookies.com*) or Suzie's organic agave sweetened spelt rice cakes. Dark 70-percent chocolate, being neutral, is also a good post–starch meal treat. In fact, dark chocolate and Hot Chocolate (see page 150) may be enjoyed after any meal, including flesh-based ones.

When you're eating a nuts/seeds/dried fruits–based meal with salad, you could enjoy any of the delicious raw treat products made by all raw bakeries. You'll find scrumptious raw brownies, raw cookies, and even raw pies! Raw Ice Cream (pages 164–167) would also be a very happy ending to a raw meal! (See appendix for extensive list of where to find these raw items.)

Desserts are important in this raw food program because they remind you that life is meant to be sweet and that you can enjoy a sweet ending after every meal if you so desire, while remaining well within the parameters of even the highest levels of the program. It's hard to complain about a diet lifestyle that allows dessert and authentic, natural sweeteners.

In terms of food combining, the Kollar cookies are a starch and as such may be enjoyed with a starch- or vegetable-based meal (not flesh or nuts/seeds/dried fruits). The chocolate is neutral and may be enjoyed after any meal! It is the perfect treat to take with you to dinner parties and even restaurants so that you can enjoy something sweet after your meal. Remember, chocolate is a stimulant and is usually accompanied by ingredients such as refined sugar, milk fat, and hydrogenated vegetable oils. However, if you are eating a very pure dark chocolate of 70 percent or more—like the ones by Green & Black and Dagoba—it will not interfere with your detoxification, and the satisfaction and pleasure it provides can make all the difference in keeping you excited about the program in the long term. Personally, I have found 70-percent chocolate extremely useful.

Raw treats are discussed in more detail later, but since they are nuts/seeds/dried fruits based, they should only be eaten as dessert after a meal consisting of raw vegetables and/or other nuts/seeds/dried fruit–based recipes. You will find that there are many delectable raw treats for you to enjoy guiltlessly.

But once again, *do not*, under any circumstances, eat a piece of fruit for dessert! As wonderful as fruit is, eating it at this time will cause all the food in your stomach to ferment and spoil, setting back the cleansing process. Of course, there are times when you just can't resist that slice of fresh apple pie. Rest assured if you practice the Raw Food Detox Diet Steps 1 to 5 about 80 percent of the time, you can freely indulge on the odd occasion. Better yet, see the recipe for Raw Cinnamon Apple-Pear Pie (page 162) and make it yourself!

If you have eaten a raw food meal such as a large raw salad and nut or dried fruit items (anything made from a nuts/seeds/dried fruits combination), you may enjoy a dessert with (or made with) bananas or dried fruit, like dates. You could make any of the raw desserts in this book or enjoy any of the raw desserts sold in many health food stores such as the Raw Bakery's raw brownies (see appendix).

Remember, this is a lifestyle, not a prison sentence. The reason this program works is because it is based on the mindset that we care about what we put into our bodies, that we want to rid ourselves of built-up toxins, and that we can enjoy nature's bounty and not be so tempted by the unnatural stimulation of processed, sugary foods.

# INFUSE YOUR BODY WITH LIVE ENZYMES

After you commit to stop poisoning your cells (and subsequently your tissues and organs) with synthetic indigestible foods and replace these foods with transition foods and quick exit meals, it's time to start hiring "workers" to do your "housecleaning."

This is where the raw foods come in. Raw foods contain something that cannot be found in any other food: *live enzymes*. Enzymes are the catalyst for every human function. We were born with the capacity to produce a great deal of enzymes and started life with a huge enzyme "bank account." However, the standard cooked American fare uses up enzymes in digestion without replacing them, and over time we become enzyme impoverished. We perceive this as a slowing metabolism. Of course our body is going to slow down if we are running low on our "workers." You'll see for yourself how your metabolism will increase when you start feeding your body live enzymes.

Returning to the concept of the enzyme bank account, when you eat uncooked plant food you are taking in large amounts of live enzymes (live enzymes mean active enzymes or enzymes that have not been destroyed by heat at temperatures of 118°F and above). The more enzymes you take in through raw plant food, the wealthier your enzyme bank account becomes. The wealthier you are in enzymes, the more fuel you will have to complete the chores that your body must do. If your body can get back to maximum production (as it did in your youth) you will suddenly find yourself living in a younger feeling body.

Here's another way to look at the importance of enzymes. We are living beings. Although no one will dispute that, our civilization consumes food that is dead—or cooked. Ask yourself, how can dead food sustain living beings without making those beings less vibrant? Eating living foods makes us more vibrant—literally "full of life."

## FOOD AND DRINK: WANTED ALIVE

To recap, the only place you will find the workers you need to detoxify your cells and restore you to a youthful state is in *uncooked plant foods and their juices*. These enzymes will happily do all your dirty work for you, scrubbing night and day while you work and sleep, but you have to get them into your system first. Since you can only get enzymes by eating uncooked plant foods, you need to figure out how often you can slip these enzymes into your meals.

As you will learn below, one of the best ways to do this is by eating nothing but fresh fruit in the morning for breakfast and by making sure you eat a sumptuous raw vegetable salad with your lunch and dinner meals. Some of my more advanced clients find that eating only uncooked plant foods until their dinner meal works very well for them. They segregate their day into two parts and know they can have a broad range of choices for a cooked dinner every night after eating a storehouse of enzymes all day. I call this "raw till dinner." They may choose to enjoy a properly combined raw or cooked meal at that time and digest it seamlessly. The added benefit to eating uncooked, enzyme-rich plant food in the predinner hours is that you avoid the fatigue that comes from eating "dead" food during the day.

The theory of eating the biggest meal early in the day is one of the major misnomers that I constantly come across. You'll see when you undertake this program that by eating lighter, enzyme-based foods in your busy working hours, you will have incredible energy. The time to eat heavier cooked foods (if you do at all) is when your working day is over and that energy is no longer needed for work. Don't take my word for it or write it off—just try it for yourself, and see if, after a few days, you aren't a convert to this approach to your daily intake. You'll also see that I have incorporated it in the upcoming menu section.

Many of you are not quite ready to go "raw till dinner" every day. But you will still see that eating the quickest exit foods early in the day and saving the heavier foods for later (ideally dinnertime) will leave you feeling much more energized during your busiest times. To best illustrate this I will borrow a term from my colleague, Gil Jacobs, who calls this way of eating "light to heavy"—meaning, going from juices to fruits to vegetables to nuts and finally to cooked food over the course of a day. Having said this, I want to emphasize that this is just a general goal. Many of you will still be eating cooked food during the day and that's just fine. As long as you are sticking closely to suggestions according to your personal Raw Transition Number (which you will determine shortly), you will be doing everything perfectly.

---

### COMING SOON TO A STORE, RESTAURANT, OR DELIVERY SERVICE NEAR YOU!

When I first started on this path it was pretty lonely. When I wanted raw desserts or a raw gourmet meal, I had to make it myself. Only a few niche raw stores like High Vibe in New York's Lower East Village (www.highvibe.com/raw) was catering to me and my "unusual" eating habits. Today, I look around and there are dozens of raw food restaurants, countless raw websites, organic delivery services, haute cuisine raw recipe books, restaurateurs, and gourmet market managers all talking about expanding their raw food offerings. The world is changing to suit those of us who are aware of the distinct connection between how we live and the food we put into our bodies. It is only going to get easier!

---

Incorporating raw foods into your diet need not be a chore. Often the term "raw foods" conjures up images of *boring* carrots and celery sticks. This is a tough image to shake, but the mouthwatering recipes in part II of this book will help you realize that raw food preparation can be even more satisfying than the foods you may be used to. Just because I am encouraging you to incorporate more raw foods into your daily diet does not mean I am suggesting that you exclusively eat raw foods.

I cannot emphasize strongly enough that an exclusively raw food diet is not the goal here. Healthy, clean cells are the goal. Raw foods do not create clean, healthy cells; the elimination of waste matter from the body does. Raw foods are extremely helpful in pulling this waste matter out of the cells, but cooked foods also play a key role in cleansing the body. Here's how: the cooked foods ensure that the cleansing is not overly aggressive. If an overweight, waste-laden person undertakes a diet that is too high in raw foods, these cleansing foods can release too much waste matter into the bloodstream and eliminative organs. If those organs are not strong enough to push those toxins out of the body or if they cannot keep up with the influx of waste that is released, the toxins will be recycled in the bloodstream, creating a condition know as *autointoxication*. The body basically retoxifies when it's unable to eliminate enough waste matter. If you follow the instructions in this book carefully and stick with your appropriate Raw Transition Number, there is no reason to be concerned about autointoxication. But to be very clear, while raw foods are an essential tool for cleaning the cells and ultimately unveiling your perfect body, they need to be understood as a vehicle to reaching that goal—not as an end unto themselves.

It takes time for the body to be clean enough to eat a 100 percent raw food diet. For those of you interested in that level of eating, I provide guidance, debunk many raw food misconceptions, and shed light on "raw done right" in part V of this book.

# THREE CORE WAYS TO FLOOD YOUR BODY WITH LIVE ENZYMES

### One: Consume only fresh fruits or fresh juices until lunchtime.

Eating only fruit in the morning is the best breakfast for a number of reasons. First, it enables you to eat one purely raw food meal in the day, which means that without much effort you could reach a minimum of 30 percent raw foods by midday. Second, since one of the keys to cleansing our bodies is to expend our internal energy on healing our bodies, we don't want to waste precious energy all day long on digesting the food we eat. With only twenty to thirty minutes transit time in the stomach, fresh fruit delivers energy to the body without wasting digestive energy. This is a win-win scenario: you get to eat but you don't have to waste energy in the stomach that would be better spent turning over new cells, healing your organs, and revving up your metabolism! The morning is also the ideal time to consume fruit since, as you now know, fruit must *only* be eaten on an empty stomach. A good rule of thumb is to wait three to four hours after a properly combined meal before eating fruit again. If you eat flesh in your meal, however, it is best not to go back to fruit again that day. I cannot stress enough that you should *never* eat fruit with any other food group or even shortly thereafter.

Morning is also the time when the body is ripe for elimination. Putting concentrated food (anything other than fresh fruits and vegetables and their juices) into the body during this time puts this elimination response (our best tool in weight loss) on hold so that the body can go to the heavily laborious task of digestion. At a time when your body is actually in a mode to help you lose excess weight (eliminate waste), don't defeat its best efforts by telling it to do something else—like digest a heavy food item or meal.

If you usually consume breakfasts of cooked, concentrated food, your body is going to expect that food tomorrow. If it does not receive that food, it is going to wonder where it is. I refer to this as "stimulation." Missing that stimulation, your body may make some growling noises or you may experience some light cramping, which is often referred to as "hunger pains." Of course, virtually no one in this country actually knows what it is to go hungry. Nonetheless, let's make it clear that you are not starving yourself or otherwise hungering. These are just signs of stimulation, and they will disappear after two to three days of eating only fruit in the morning.

You should not feel light-headed because you will be getting plenty of fruit sugar into your bloodstream. Mentally you should feel very clear, while physically light and energetic. If you feel light-headed you are most likely not eating enough fruit. Feel free to eat as much fruit as you need. You might eat a cantaloupe at eight o'clock in the morning, a box of strawberries at nine, a couple of bananas at ten, and then some sliced pineapple at eleven. This would certainly be well within the range of a typical Raw Food Detox breakfast. Some of you are thinking that this sounds like more than you could ever eat. Others of you can imagine yourselves easily going through this much fruit before lunch. Find the amount that works for you, and be aware that it might vary from day to day.

## Two: Devour Green Lemonade

If I were to tell you that there is something that you can drink that literally infuses your body with millions of enzymes, keeps your immune system strong year-round, offers unparalleled protection against osteoporosis, and tastes highly refreshing and filling, would you want some? It's called Green Lemonade, and I don't know a single successful raw foodist who does not drink some variation of this recipe (see recipe below) as *the foundation* of their Raw Food Diet.

It's a fact: nothing is more live-enzyme rich than freshly extracted vegetable juice. Ounce for ounce it is the most enzyme-loaded, easily absorbable form of nutrition available on the planet today. Unfortunately, when most people think of vegetable juice, they typically picture canned V-8 or, worse still, nauseating shots of wheatgrass juice! I'm never surprised when, at the first mention of green juice, my clients cringe. What they don't know yet is that there is a way to make vegetable juice surprisingly tasty and borderline addictive! I call this "Green Lemonade." Try it! You'll love it!

# Green Lemonade

**MAKES 1 SERVING**

1 head romaine lettuce or celery

5 to 6 stalks kale (any type)

1 to 2 apples (as needed for sweetness—I recommend organic Fuji)

1 whole organic lemon (you don't have to peel it)

1 to 2 inches fresh ginger (optional)

Process the vegetables in a juicer (please see information about juicing below). Pour into a large glass, and drink! Notice how the lemon really cuts out the "green" taste that most people try to avoid.

You may use any greens in place of the romaine and kale—like celery, chard, collards, spinach, cucumber, and so forth—as long as there are some dark leafy greens in there, too! This recipe shows a way to keep it simple with just two types of greens.

For best results, enjoy Green Lemonade on an empty stomach. It's perfect in the morning thirty minutes on either side of fresh fruit, or in the afternoon at least three hours after a properly combined lunch, or thirty minutes before dinner. But it's not a good idea to drink it with meals. Sipping a bit of liquid (like wine) is fine, but liquid dilutes the digestive juices that we depend on for optimum digestion. The goal is to start by drinking approximately 12 ounces of Green Lemonade each day. Gradually work your way up to 24 to 40 ounces each day (at the highest Personal Transition level). Some is better than none. You cannot drink too much of it—as long as it's consumed separately from food.

**Why juice the vegetables instead of eating them?**

Imagine chopping all the above ingredients into a bowl and eating them. It would take quite a lot of time and particularly a lot of chewing! However, by juicing them we can ingest the quintessential organic water, chlorophyll, and enzymes from heaping mounds of romaine lettuce, kale, cucumber, celery, and other greens in just minutes, without expending any digestive energy. In addition to getting innumerable amounts of enzymes from drinking vegetable juices, there also are enzymes trapped deep inside the fibers of fresh vegetables that we can't absorb through normal digestion but that can be released by a juicer.

**Is a juicer different from a blender?**

Yes! A juicer separates the juice from the fiber of the vegetables, leaving you with only the pure organic water from the vegetables. If you put the above ingredients into a blender, it will mix the items together while retaining the fiber, and you'll end up with a blended soup. While blenders are very useful for making sauces, soups, shakes, and blended salads, you'll need an actual juicer to make vegetable juice.

While there are a number of excellent juice bars in cities across the United States, it's great to have your own juicer. There are so many juicers on the market today, but the Breville is far and away the easiest to use when you are juicing lots of greens. You can order a Breville juicer at www.highvibe.com/raw. Look for a juicer that extracts the pulp, as it will allow you to make more juice without having to stop to clean it, and it can handle greens better than one that holds the pulp in. Since you will mainly be juicing greens, this is very important.

### Why would I want to separate the juice from the fiber?

When the juice is separated from the fiber we can ingest much more of the organic water from the vegetables because the bulk of the fiber does not get in the way and fill us up. This organic water that is extracted from the vegetables contains all of the vitamins, minerals, and enzymes from the plant. Fiber is nothing more than roughage. That's not to say that fiber is not important—of course it is! But you are going to be getting so much fiber in a raw food–based diet that you don't need to worry about missing it in your juice. Further, because there is no fiber in the juice, your body will not waste energy on digestion. The enzymes go straight to cellular level to do their work. Remember, when enzymes can go straight into the cells they can go to work cleaning out the rubbish and making you leaner and healthier!

### Did you know that green juices are pure organic hydration and oxygenation?

Organic hydration describes water derived from plant sources (like green vegetable juice) instead of from a spring, well, or faucet. The minerals that you get from vegetables and their juices can be easily absorbed as opposed to those from mineral water. Minerals from mineral water and sea salts do not get absorbed into the cells and can actually have the adverse effect of leaching minerals from the body (consider the effect on your bones).

These green juices provide perfect cellular hydration and will take the place of drinking glasses of water. You *will not* need to drink the regulation eight to ten glasses of water each day when you are on this program. You will be juicing and ingesting a hydrating diet of fresh fruits and vegetables, leaving your cells with little to no additional water requirements.

The only reason the average American needs so much water is because his/her diet con-

---

### THE CARROT TRICK:

Keep bags of organic carrots in the fridge for predinner munchies. Not only are they sweet and delicious but they are also very hydrating after a long day. You could eat an entire 2-pound bag of carrots while you're unwinding, reading the mail, or putting your kids to bed. This would take the edge off your appetite, nourish your body with organic minerals and enzymes, and give your children a good example of a smart snack.

## WHAT IS A SALAD, REALLY?

Often when I first ask a client what she (or he) is eating I hear, "Oh, I mostly just eat salads." But this person has come to see me for a reason: she has 30 or 40 pounds to lose and may suffer from chronic asthma. She cannot possibly be living on salads! I proceed to ask her exactly what goes into her salads. At first she typically starts listing raw vegetables. If at this point I have not gotten the details that she may inadvertently be withholding, I'll probe deeper: "What about cheese? Do you put any corn, beans, chicken, or croutons in your salads?" Inevitably, she will respond, "Oh yes, a little blue cheese, some chicken, maybe some raisins or chick peas." Ah ha! Folks, this is not a salad—it's a tossed meal! For our purposes, the term "salad" means one thing: raw vegetables!

sists exclusively of nonhydrated foods. For example, if you eat a bagel for breakfast, you need water to offset the density of the food. But enjoy half of a watermelon instead and you'll be fully hydrated! Do you get it? The rules for the average American dieter are completely different from the rules on this program because you are eating (and drinking) foods that your body is made to eat—not the synthetic diet that is crippling our nation from the inside out!

Also keep in mind that oxygen is one of the components of water and is the essential requirement for cell life. Without oxygen, cells will die. By consistently infusing our bodies with hydrating, oxygen-rich raw foods and juices, we ensure that quantities of oxygen—above and beyond what we take in through normal breathing—are encouraging and nourishing healthy cells.

### What about bottled vegetable juices like Odwalla and Fresh Samantha?

Although some of these juices appear to be fresh pressed, they are not. Just as in the case of bottled fruit juices, the above mentioned brands have been pasteurized, which kills the live enzymes. Bottled juices do not count as green juices for our purposes, and should be avoided. However, if your grocer bottles freshly squeezed juices (orange, grapefruit, carrot, etc.) as many grocers do nowadays, these would be fine for you to include as part of your "raw quota" and regular menu.

### Where can I find freshly extracted juice and/or Green Lemonade if I don't want to make my own?

A juice bar is a good place to go, but be careful not to assume that anything you get at a juice bar is good for you. For example, there are many chains of juice bars that mainly make blended smoothies with frozen, sugared fruits, soy, or frozen yogurt. You can usually get a glass of carrot juice or a shot of wheatgrass at these places, but be very careful ordering the blended drinks—unless you are specific about what goes into them.

### What about those green powders?

Green powder supplements are not the same as fresh green juices. Primarily they are lacking in the organic hydration. They are being reconstituted in water instead of the vegetables themselves. But they are helpful when you're traveling, and they are better than nothing.

### Three: don't eat your cooked food until you've eaten your raw food.

Let's face it, how many of you are going to eat your raw vegetable salad after your bowl of pasta? You'll enjoy and digest your raw food better if you eat it as the first course of your repast. Make a great big raw vegetable salad with a stunning raw dressing (see recipe section). Enjoy this salad as a staple before you eat any cooked foods. Then, if you are planning on a cooked dish, enjoy it! Eating the salad first will ensure that you make at least half of your meal all-raw.

# YOU NEED TO TAKE THE GARBAGE OUT!

What would happen if you started cleaning your house but left the garbage in random heaps throughout it? Your house wouldn't actually get clean, and soon those heaps would make their way around the whole house again. It would be a wasted effort all in all. Likewise, if you do all the hard work to clean your body but leave the debris in heaps around the eliminative organs without ensuring they get fully eliminated, they are simply going to resettle in your cells again. This goes back to the principle of autointoxication that we discussed earlier. To avoid this, your organs need some extra help to eliminate the waste you've collected. This is the time to call in "the waste management specialists."

As you cleanse your body, the waste is directed to your five major eliminative organs for discarding; these include the skin, kidneys, colon, spleen, and liver. The waste matter you've drawn up through the detox diet will be processed through all of these organs as part of your "local waste management system." If you are young and strong, your body will manage much of this waste seamlessly. But if you are over thirty and in poor condition, there are several things that you can do to help this process along. While you might not be inclined to try all of the following ideas, I would highly recommend that you take on at least a couple of them. The more you can do to help with the elimination of this matter, the more quickly you will get your desired results. Remember: Waste = Weight!

# WASTE MANAGEMENT SPECIALIST TIP #1: EMPLOY GRAVITY METHOD COLONIC HYDRATION

In an ideal world, the colon would eliminate the residue from the food that is digested in the intestines after complete processing. If this were true for you, you would move your bowels five times each day for every three meals and two snacks that you consume, per the standard American diet. Do you move your bowels five times? I didn't think so. Do you move your bowels once a day? Well, that's helpful, but not nearly enough. Are you chronically constipated or do you struggle with IBS or other digestive disorders? Many of you do, as I've seen in my practice.

Think for a moment about what happens when you do not eliminate the waste from your meal. Whatever is not eliminated gets baked into your cells and into your intestines at 98.6°F (that's basically the temperature of a dehydrator). This matter gets further cooked into your cells over time and can remain in your body indefinitely, slowing down your body's overall physical performance. Combine this backup in your colon with the waste that you have drawn up through your detoxification, and you can imagine how helpful it would be to have this waste gently and safely removed.

### What is a colonic?

A colonic is a method of removing waste matter from the colon. In the case of a gravity method colonic, you simply lie on your left side and allow the trained colon therapist to insert the metal instrument (called a "speculum") about a quarter-inch into your rectum. This speculum is connected to tubing which is connected to a tank of water that rests about three feet above your feet. The therapist allows the water to gently flow through the tubing into your colon while the waste-heavy water moves out of you through the "exit" tubing and into the septic system. After a brief time on your left side, you move on to your back as the session continues. Your colon therapist may massage your midsection to encourage the body to release waste in various areas of your colon. The whole session lasts forty-five to sixty minutes.

### How often should colonics be administered?

This is a very personal decision. The best rule of thumb I can give you is to start by going about once a month. As you incorporate more of the principles of this book, you might want to go more frequently for a while to ensure the waste you're drawing up leaves the body promptly. This will leave you feeling better and leaner with every session. You'll find the balance that suits your lifestyle. Colonics become more important as your diet becomes more raw. The more aggressively you cleanse (through consuming raw foods), the more waste you will draw up for removal. If your body is managing this waste well through increased bowel activity, and if you are not experiencing any detox symptoms like skin eruptions, headaches, flu-like symptoms, joint pain, and so forth, then you don't need to have the colonics. The detox symptoms show that there's waste that's not getting out through the basic means. This is when colonics save the day! Those of you who find a top-rate colon therapist and embrace this "waste management" method will quickly see how regular treatments can transform your body and make you feel like a kid again in a fraction of the time that it would otherwise take.

### Are there any drawbacks to colonics?

There are no drawbacks to a properly administered gravity method colonic. However, as with all things, there are top-rate versus second-rate specialists and methods. The very best method of colonic hydration is called the gravity method, which employs the force of gravity to move the water into your body. This method also employs a stainless steel instrument as opposed to the less preferable plastic, disposable one, which is not as gentle on the rectum.

### Where can I get a colonic and how much does it cost?

Check the appendix for a listing of colon therapists near you. Sessions range from $50 to $110. Or call the Wood Hygienic Institute at 407-933-0009 and ask them for a certified colon therapist in your area. (Note: Do not eat three hours prior to treatment and try to have a green juice or green salad directly following your treatment.)

## WASTE MANAGEMENT SPECIALIST TIP #2: FAMILIARIZE YOURSELF WITH AN ENEMA KIT.

An enema is the next best thing to getting a colonic. In this case, you would want to purchase a Cara enema kit at www.highvibe.com/raw, which uses fresh water. The Fleet-style enema brand is not recommended as it contains chemicals. However, if this is all you can find, empty the Fleet of its contents and simply fill it with fresh water and administer per the instructions on the package. (In fact, you can use any two-quart enema kit and fill it with bottled water.) An enema kit is useful to keep around even if you do get regular colonics. It's great to take with you when you travel or to use just to clear a headache or other symptom, instead of going in for a colonic. The Cara enema kit also uses a gravity method and is very easy to self-administer.

### How to Self-administer an Enema

1. Assemble the enema bag per the instructions on the box.

2. Fill the enema bag with water (filtered or bottled water is preferable).

3. Release the clamp on the tubing and allow a little water to flow into the sink for just a moment to release the air and reclamp.

4. Place the hook of the enema bag on a towel rack or on something steady about three feet above the ground.

5. Place a towel underneath you (on top of a carpet or rug so it's soft) and lie down on your left side.

6. Place a bit of lubrication (butter or olive oil works well) on the plastic tip that you will insert into your rectum.

7. Gently insert the lubricated plastic tip about one inch into your rectum.

8. Release the clamp and allow the water to flow. Allow yourself to take in just enough water to make you feel comfortably full. Never force yourself to take in too much water—there is no benefit to doing that.

9. Try to hold the water in until you feel you must release it.

10. When you're ready to release the water, sit on the toilet and release.

11. Continue this process for as long as waste matter is leaving your system.

12. Wash your kit thoroughly with warm water and soap, and either dry it and put it away or let it air dry.

13. You should feel much lighter and energized afterward!

### Tips for Taking an Enema

■ If you only release dirty water and no waste matter, stop the process. You are only backing the waste deeper into the colon. Wait a day or so and try again.

■ If you are removing waste, continue taking the enema until you stop releasing waste.

- Massage your midsection gently in a clockwise motion if you are able. This will encourage a more effective release.

- If you are traveling, try to use just a little water at first to see if the matter comes out easily. You don't want to back yourself up on the road.

- Never force yourself to hold more water than you should. If the water hits matter, you will not easily take in more. This matter will be released with the small amount of water but may be pushed back with too much water.

- Always elevate your feet on a stool (more details below) when releasing the water and waste.

## WASTE MANAGEMENT SPECIALIST TIP #3: USE A STOOL FOR YOUR STOOL

Now you must really think I have a one-track mind, but the elimination of waste matter from your largest eliminative organ is so fundamental to your success that the topic is bound to keep popping up!

Throughout time humans have moved their bowels in a squatting position. With the advent of the modern-day toilet, we started sitting—and therefore shifting the position of our rectum during this key natural process. The sitting posture takes our rectum out of ideal alignment, which results in less effective bowel movements. This in turn creates more waste matter buildup, impaction, constipation, and putrefaction in the intestines. All of this could be relieved in large part simply by putting your rectum back into proper alignment; prop your feet up between six to eighteen inches off the floor. You don't even need to buy anything special. Your bathroom waste basket (now that gives new meaning to the term) would probably work, as would a foot stool or filing box. Be creative. But just be sure to have something close at hand and use it every time you need to move your bowels. For those of you suffering from constipation, just start your day by sitting in this position and imagine the waste leaving your system. After a few days, you'll be able to stimulate better movements just by thinking about it!

# WASTE MANAGEMENT SPECIALIST TIP #4:
# DRY BRUSHING AND MASSAGE THERAPY

Did you know that you release between 2 to 5 pounds of toxins through your skin every day? This means your skin—the largest organ in your body—is the second most powerful elimination force in the body. One of the best ways to take advantage of this opportunity to release more toxins is to use a natural bristle skin brush every day. This brush, which you can find in your local health food store, can literally brush away waste from the skin. At about $8, a natural bristle dry brush is one of the best kept beauty secrets around. One brush should last you several months and can be cleaned with soap and warm water after every three to four uses. (I recommend the Yerba Prima body brush available at www.highvibe.com/raw.)

Dry brushing on a regular basis lightens the burden of excess waste on your liver and spleen. The skin is the largest organ in the body and is key to delivering oxygen to your cells. It's easy to forget that skin breathes. Dry brushing lifts off all the waste matter and allows the skin to take in much more oxygen, as well as throw off more waste matter. Furthermore, dry brushing stimulates the lymphatic system, which moves the waste through the body to eliminative organs and lymphatic drainage areas. By stroking the body with the dry brush and focusing on these lymphatic drainage regions you will increase the efficiency of the whole lymphatic system!

## How to use a natural bristle body brush

Remove your clothes, then take the brush off its handle for easier mobility. Starting with the soles of the feet, begin dry brushing the body using long upward strokes. Brush from the ankles to the calves, concentrating on the area behind the knees. Then brush from the knees to the groin, the thighs, and the buttocks. If you're a woman, make *circular* strokes around your thighs and buttocks to help mobilize fat stores (it's great for cellulite). Then brush the torso (avoiding the breasts). Finally, make long strokes from the wrists to the shoulders and underarms. This should take no more than five minutes and will leave you feeling totally invigorated! The best times to brush are in the morning before exercising or showering, or before retiring at night.

## Massage therapy (or self-massage)

This is another great way to help remove waste matter by supporting the flow of lymphatic fluid through the body. And for those of you who believe in increasing the flow of chi in your body, massage therapy is great for revitalizing the body and lifting away its stagnant energies.

## WASTE MANAGEMENT SPECIALIST TIP #5: BOUNCE LIKE A KID!

Do you remember what it was like to jump on a trampoline? As a kid it probably never occurred to you that being buoyant was especially good for you—you did it just because it felt good. It so happens that jumping on a trampoline or a mini-trampoline (called a rebounder) is possibly the single best exercise on the planet. Rebounding literally squeezes the waste matter from our cells as we bounce effortlessly for just a short time. It is ideal for circulation and great for toning the whole body. But best of all, it supports the lymphatic system by internally massaging the lymph drainage points and carrying the lymph fluid through the body more efficiently.

You can buy a cheap rebounder at most sporting goods stores, but it may not stand the test of time. I recommend Needak rebounders (about $250 at www.highvibe.com/raw) or try to find an inexpensive used one.

## WASTE MANAGEMENT SPECIALIST TIP #6: DEEP BREATHING

Lest we forget, our lungs are also an eliminative organ. Every time we exhale we are releasing waste matter through the breath. However, we typically take such shallow breaths that we hardly maximize the cleaning ability of this organ. Take advantage of moments in the day when you can focus on your breath and inhale and exhale deeply to maximize oxygen intake and waste removal. And hey, there's the added benefit of feeling positively zen-like!

## WASTE MANAGEMENT SPECIALIST TIP #7: INVERSIONS

In yoga talk "inversion" means a position in which your head is below your feet—as in a handstand, headstand, shoulder stand, and so forth. Anyone who has not been properly educated in inversions should not undertake this type of yogic posture. However, beginners can create the beneficial effect of inversions simply by elevating the feet and/or pelvis to increase blood flow to the organs and get fresh oxygenated blood to the brain. All forms of exercise do this by pumping blood through the body at an increased rate, but inversions deliver the uniquely purifying experience of reversing gravity on the body, thereby recharging it on so many levels. If you are skilled at inversions, I highly recommend them as a regular part of your cleansing lifestyle.

# WASTE MANAGEMENT SPECIALIST TIP #8: SWEAT IT OUT AND LET THE SUNSHINE IN!

Going back to your skin's eliminative powers, you must not overlook the importance of sweat as a carrier of waste matter. Whether you sweat by exercising, sitting in a sauna or steam room, or working in your backyard, sweating is a key waste elimination method. The more you sweat, the more waste you will help your body release.

While a traditional sauna is better than nothing, an infrared sauna is superior. Infrared energy is also known as radiant energy—the kind of energy our sun produces. It is a powerful tool for removing deeply lodged toxins, including heavy metals like mercury, from the tissues. While being many times more effective than a traditional sauna, it is not as hot so you will enjoy a much more comfortable experience and be able to stay in longer. With its excellent ability to draw out old wastes from the cells and tissues, many people report a significant reduction in cellulite. Starting around $2,000 for a two-person unit, infrared saunas are not for everyone. (You might consider getting together with a couple of friends and sharing a unit). However, those who can afford it will benefit and enjoy it tremendously. To learn more about the benefits of an infrared sauna, check out the link on my website, www.TheRawFoodDetoxDiet.com

Sunshine is also a highly underrated cleanser. It has the ability to reach inside our cells and pull impurities to the surface. Sweating in the early morning or late afternoon sun is ideal. Sunbathe as often as you can in those safe-sun hours (before 10:00 A.M. or after 4:00 P.M.). Instead of putting clogging SPF protection on your skin for these short, safe bouts of sun, wear a hat and/or light clothing. There is no reason that we as a society cannot learn to appreciate and respect the sun. The sun is literally the light of our lives and source of all energy on Earth. Yet after years of excessive sunbathing in the heat of the day, we have come to shun it. If we respect the sun and enjoy it in reasonable doses, we have no need to fear it or apply toxic skin creams that may become harmful when combined with the sun's rays, or even make their way into our bloodstream.

# DETERMINE YOUR RAW FOOD TRANSITION NUMBER

This is the most important tool for getting this program right! It is critical to personalize your weight loss and rejuvenating experience based on your unique health and weight history. Take the following test to discover your personal Raw Food Transition Number. This number will determine precisely how you should adapt the Raw Food Detox Diet steps in the first month and how you'll progress over time.

For each question, answer yes, no, or somewhat.

1. Were you raised on sugared cereals, "TV dinners," and fast food (regardless of your current age and lifestyle)?

2. Are you a smoker or have you smoked for over eight years?

3. Are meat, potatoes, white flour, animal fats, cooked oils, and white sugar a part of your normal eating pattern?

4. Do you have a history of drug use or have you taken birth control and/or other hormones, steroids, or undergone chemotherapy?

5. Do you have a history of IBS, constipation, colitis, or other bowel/digestive disorders?

    **6.** Are you over forty years old?

    **7.** Are you between 20 and 30 pounds overweight?

    **8.** Are you more than 80 pounds overweight?

    **9.** Do you suffer from asthma, bronchial infections, chronic colds and flus, or other mucosal conditions?

    **10.** Do you have a sedentary lifestyle?

    **11.** Are dairy products (cheese, milk, yogurt, cottage cheese, etc.) a mainstay of your diet?

    **12.** Do you eat animal protein more than four times a week?

    **13.** Do you eat soy products on a regular basis (soy milk, tofu, soy chips, soy meats, etc.)?

    **14.** Do you consume more than three sodas (diet or otherwise) each week?

    **15.** Do you suffer from liver disorder, acne, psoriasis, or other skin disorders?

Calculating your Raw Food Transition Number: For every "yes" answer, give yourself 2 points; for every "sometimes" answer, give yourself 1 point; for every "no" answer, give yourself zero points.

# IF YOU SCORED 20+ POINTS, YOU ARE A LEVEL 5

You are health challenged. You always thought a salad was coleslaw or that green and red stuff on a burger. You feel heavy and tired most of the time, and you just want to start losing weight. But you've been on diets before and you know where they typically leave you. It's time to introduce you to the pleasures of raw foods—some fresh fruit for breakfast, a bag of baby carrots as an afternoon snack, a delicious salad, and your first glass of Green Lemonade!

    **Your parameters for cleansing:** Embrace a daily diet of 75 percent raw foods. See page 71 for your one-week sample menu plan.

    **Choose your battles:** Cutting out coffee and condiments and eating organic foods are not the battles you should be fighting. Your strategy consists of following the Raw Food Detox Diet Steps #1 and #2.

Your success hinges on finding the pleasure in these transition foods and quick exit foods. Think about what you can have, not what you shouldn't. Putting together enough menu ideas and restaurant options from part II of this book will enable you to feel really good and excited about your food experiences.

**As a Level 5, will I see any benefits from making just a few small changes?**

The answer is a resounding yes! One of the most important things I try to convey to my clients is how valuable "baby steps" can be when moving toward this way of eating. First, taking baby steps means taking off the pressure, so burnout and boredom are not likely. Second, it gently initiates the body in detoxification, so you're not likely to experience uncomfortable symptoms. Third, taking things slowly helps to ensure you will stick with this Raw Food Detox Diet long term. People looking for a quick fix tend to go right back to their old habits as soon as they see results.

If you would like to take it slowly, I would recommend starting with just one of the following principles and incorporating more of them over time. Each one of these principles will produce terrific benefits on their own:

1. Focus on fruit alone as your morning meal.

2. Eliminate all foods that contain simple carbohydrates: white flour, white potatoes, and white sugar.

3. Focus on keeping starch foods and protein foods separate.

4. Focus on increasing your percentage of raw food intake to 70 percent or more.

5. Begin to eliminate dairy products.

# IF YOU SCORED 14 TO 19 POINTS, YOU ARE A LEVEL 4

You and your body are ready for a change. You may or may not have the discipline to take on a drastic dietary change, but you're at the starting gate and you are certainly willing to try it for a couple of weeks. You're hoping this will be the diet that finally makes it happen, but you've had your hopes dashed before. Still, unadulterated foods makes real intuitive sense to you and you've seen photographs of celebrities who've been radically transformed by this all-natural approach to foods. Your doctor has likely warned you about what could happen if you don't change your diet to start preventing disease. You have a lot at stake, including your happiness. You feel that, if you were just told exactly what to do to get results, you could do it.

**Your parameters for cleansing:** Embrace a daily diet of 80 to 85 percent raw foods. This is not as difficult as it may sound. In addition to eating an all-fruit/vegetable juice breakfast, all you need to do is make sure that half of your lunch and half of your dinner consist of raw plant food—like a large fresh vegetable salad. See page 74 for your one-week sample menu plan.

**Choose your battles:** Don't be concerned about the relative minutiae of eliminating your morning cup of "Joe" or ensuring you only eat organic produce. Your battle is in working to get only real foods into your system. Focus on Raw Food Detox Steps #1 and #2 and begin to incorporate Step #3.

Your success hinges on being prepared for every lifestyle scenario. You must plan for your engagements and your activities by having a strategy in place (i.e. taking raw nuts and dried fruits or bananas to your son's afternoon soccer game, or finding out what your mother is serving for brunch so you can suggest bringing a salad and some sweet potatoes, if there's nothing on her menu for you).

# IF YOU SCORED 8 TO 13 POINTS, YOU ARE A LEVEL 3

The idea of cleansing your body holds great appeal to you and you're ready to make a fully conscious effort to eat mostly cleansing meals. You like to have some flexibility with your dinners, but you already feel that eating this way gives you more energy during the day and is surprisingly satisfying. In a short time, you notice a new-found equilibrium in your day-to-day regime by eating mostly uncooked, plant-based meals. Your bowel activity has profoundly increased and you're really making the connection between your weight, health, and the elimination of garbage from your system. You've had your fair share of "cleansing responses" (symptoms like headaches, acne, and indigestion) but the worst is behind you. You can maintain this level of eating for a lifetime and lose virtually all of your excess weight. But, when the time is right, you'll most likely progress to the next level. If Level 3 feels this good, you can just imagine how wonderful Level 2 is going to feel!

**Your parameters for raw foods:** Embrace a daily diet of 85 to 90 percent raw foods—essentially eating "raw till dinner" every day (six to eight cooked meals per week). See page 77 for your one-week sample menu plan.

**Choose your battles:** Your challenges are against the random temptations like cookies in the office, or friends and family pressuring you to eat as they do. This is the stage at which you begin to reclaim your power and do what's good for you—not what makes everybody around you happy. This is the time to start challenging periphery habits like your daily cup(s) of coffee and increasing the quality of your fruits and vegetables. Try to make buying organic produce a standard practice when and where you can, particularly when buying bananas, avocados, and leafy greens. Hone in on perfecting your food combinations, eating a lighter lunch (raw when possible) and a heavier dinner (high-quality cooked and raw foods).

Your success hinges on discovering how delicious and filling your all-raw meals can be. Try at least two new raw recipes a week.

## IF YOU SCORED 4 TO 7 POINTS, YOU ARE A LEVEL 2

You are now ready for the second most advanced level. Uncooked plant foods taste good to you—particularly because you've learned some of the very simple recipes in this book and found them to be positively stunning! It is easy for you to eat "raw till dinner" every day of the week. You're used to taking good care of yourself. (Beware of reaching this level prematurely, just because you think you've been so "good" over the years and you know so much about health. You'll know if it's too soon by your body's response.) If you do indeed belong here as a Level 2, you will not judge yourself. You genuinely love your cleansing meals, and when you don't, you eat what you want to eat. You feel comfortable eating only uncooked plant foods during the day because you know you can have any high-quality, properly combined cooked meal you desire for dinner. You have also mastered making raw dressings, dishes, and ice creams so that you never feel deprived when you eat raw. You no longer count calories or fat grams and you can easily see eating this way for the rest of your life.

**Your parameters for raw foods:** Embrace a daily diet of 90 to 95 percent uncooked plant foods (three to five meals a week could be cooked). See page 80 for your one-week sample menu plan. Now you're really playing ball.

**Choose your battles:** If you are feeling sluggish or struggling at this level, it probably isn't the right level for you. Don't be afraid to go back to Level 3 or 4 for as long as it takes to prepare yourself for Level 2.

Your success hinges on consistently expanding your raw recipe repertoire, ordering or buying plenty of "raw treats" for your all-raw dinners, ensuring that you are paying attention to your elimination needs, and making sure that your bowel activity is keeping up with your detoxification response.

# IF YOU SCORED LESS THAN 3 POINTS, YOU ARE A LEVEL 1

You are ready for the most advanced level, which means that virtually all but one or maybe two dinners each week will be raw. While you may eat all-raw for days or even weeks at a time, you may enjoy going "off the rails" for dinner whenever you desire to do so. You know that it is easiest on your system not to eat cooked dinners two days in a row, but there will be times when you do it anyway, like if you're on vacation. You find it easy to stick to this level of the program because your cellular health is now so superior that you do not crave the foods you ate before. You know that when those cravings for heavy foods kick in, it simply means that there is some impaction in your system and one good session with a quality colon therapist will set you right. (Note: This is a highly advanced level that does not work for everyone. Very few people are ready to start at this level.)

**Your parameters for raw foods:** Embrace a weekly diet of 98+ percent raw foods. This means that out of twenty-one meals each week, only one meal would be cooked. See page 84 for your one-week sample menu plan.

**Choose your battles:** The great news is that once you've been cleansing at this level for a while, the battles are few. You've faced and slain the biggest dragons in the preceding levels. My advice at this level (as well as at preceding levels) is to make it as easy as possible for you to get fresh, organic produce.

Your success hinges on commitment. This level is not for someone who eats out frequently (although it can be done) or someone who is not ready to commit deeply to eating this way in the long term. This level is not for everyone, but for a true Level 1, it is sheer body paradise!

# HOW TO DETERMINE WHEN YOU'RE READY TO MOVE UP A LEVEL

There is a very simple test to determine if you are ready to move up a level. Try a week at the level you are aiming for. See how you feel. If you are satisfied by the foods and your eliminations keep pace with what you eat, you can proceed. I recommend spending at least one month at each level before moving up. You can always go back a level for awhile if you feel it's necessary. This need not be a linear process. Do what feels right to you. For instance, a Level 1 or 2 may prefer to go back a level in the winter in order to include more cooked foods (like steamed vegetables, carrots, and sweet potatoes) for dinner, then go back to eating almost 100 percent raw in the spring.

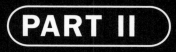

# MENUS FOR ALL RAW FOOD TRANSITION NUMBERS

# TIPS ON USING
# THE MENU SECTION

- You do not have to eat everything suggested.

- Days are completely interchangeable.

- Always wait a full three hours before switching food categories—such as eating an avocado sandwich at lunch to having raisins as an afternoon snack—because it is critical that each meal/food leave the stomach before the next category of food is taken in to ensure optimum digestion and detoxification.

- The menus may be followed to the letter or just used as a guide. As long as you are following the steps outlined in part I, you can customize your daily menus accordingly.

- If you don't like something that is listed, you may substitute it with a dish that you do like as long as it is for the same mealtime.

- If you are on a tight budget, see page 184 for inexpensive meal ideas to substitute for any lunch or dinner dish.

- Refer to the section on Eating Out in part IV so that you can easily substitute a Raw Food Detox meal when dining out. (That section also includes suggestions for fast-food venues.)

- Rarely will you see a portion size listed in the menu section. This is because raw foods and cooked quick exit foods can be eaten in fairly liberal quantities.

Whether you have a small or large appetite, you should be able to eat to satisfaction. However, you never want to overeat because that creates as much of a drain on your "detox energy" as would a poorly combined meal. When you come to mealtime with an enormous appetite, eat generous amounts of raw salads and soups first, instead of filling up on the nut/dried fruit concoctions, raw treats, and cooked starches. But you can eat hearty quantities of all the foods listed in the recipe section regardless of calorie or sugar content. Tap into your own sense of appropriate sizes and, if you are honest with yourself, you will know the difference between eating heartily and bingeing!

# DETOX TRANSITION LEVEL 5

**Personal Profile** A Level 5 is typically more than 80 pounds overweight, over forty years old, and usually has family members who suffer from heart disease or cancer. A Level 5 has a history of eating in fast-food restaurants and consuming processed foods regularly. He or she may also have a history of yo-yo dieting and drinking lots of diet soda. Another example of a Level 5 would include a person who is not particularly overweight but has undergone extensive drug therapy, like IVF, chemo, steroids, or recreational drugs.

## The Raw Food Detox Diet Menu for Level 5

(Italicized recipes are in this book)

> *If you have been on low-carb diets, you may be worried about the sugar and starch content of this daily menu. As you will see, the sprouted grain bread products and crackers are so easily digested, and the fruit sugars and carrots are so hydrating and alive, that they will all work together to help the weight come off while leaving you feeling utterly satisfied. You're just going to have to allow yourself to think beyond the calories and carb grams to see the results for yourself!*

### Day 1
**Upon rising:** A piece of fresh fruit
**Breakfast** (at least 20 minutes later): 2 slices sprouted grain toast or 4 Ak-Mak crackers

with ½ a fresh avocado sliced on top and 3 celery stalks (to help carry it through the body)

**Lunch:** Fresh raw vegetable salad with *Liquid Gold Elixir* salad dressing, *Avocado-Vegetable Sandwich*

**Snack:** 1 bag of baby carrots

**Dinner:** *Quick Guacamole Salad, Whole Wheat Lasagna*

**Dessert:** 3 Kollar cookies or ⅓ bar Dagoba 75-percent chocolate

## Day 2

**Upon rising:** A piece of fresh fruit

**Breakfast** (at least 20 minutes later): 2 slices sprouted grain toast or 4 Ak-Mak crackers with fresh avocado slices and 3 celery stalks

**Lunch:** *Carrot–Sweet Potato Bisque* or any Taste Adventure brand soup, 2 slices sprouted grain toast (organic butter and raw honey optional), large, fresh raw vegetable salad with *Liquid Gold Elixir* salad dressing

**Snack** (3 hours later): Fresh carrot juice, 2 bananas or 8 to 20 ounces *Green Lemonade*

**Dinner:** Green salad, *Endive Bruschetta*, 1 bowl kamut pasta topped with steamed broccoli and Seeds of Change pasta sauce

**Dessert:** 3 Kollar cookies or *Hot Chocolate* and ⅓ bar Dagoba 75-percent chocolate

## Day 3

**Upon rising:** A piece of fresh fruit

**Breakfast** (at least 20 minutes later): 2 slices sprouted grain toast with fresh avocado slices and 3 celery stalks

**Lunch:** Large, fresh raw vegetable salad, *Liquid Gold Elixir* salad dressing, 1 cup brown rice (organic butter and Celtic sea salt optional), 2 cups steamed vegetables

**Snack** (3 hours later): Fresh fruit as desired or 8 to 20 ounces *Green Lemonade*

**Dinner:** *Classic Chopped Salad, Maple-Glazed Salmon*, steamed vegetables as desired

**Dessert:** ⅓ bar Dagoba 75-percent chocolate or up to ⅓ package Alta Dena raw cheddar-style goat cheese

## Day 4

**Upon rising:** A piece of fresh fruit

**Breakfast** (at least 20 minutes later): Sprouted grain toast with fresh avocado slices and 3 celery stalks

**Lunch:** Large, fresh raw vegetable salad, *Raw Ranch Dressing*, 2 sweet potatoes, 4 Ak-Mak crackers (organic butter optional)

**Snack** (3 to 4 hours later): 1 bag of baby carrots, 1 small box of raisins, 4 ounces of your favorite raw nuts

**Dinner** (3 to 4 hours later): Large, fresh raw vegetable salad (goat cheese optional), organic chicken (baked, rotisserie, or roasted), 1 to 2 cups steamed vegetables

**Dessert:** ⅓ bar Dagoba 75-percent chocolate

## Day 5

**Upon rising:** A piece of fresh fruit

**Breakfast** (at least 20 minutes later): Sprouted grain toast with fresh avocado slices and 3 celery stalks

**Lunch:** Large, fresh raw vegetable salad with *Liquid Gold Elixir* salad dressing, *Hurgry-Girl Omelet*, steamed vegetables as desired

**Snack** (at least 2 hours later): Fresh carrot juice or *Green Lemonade*

**Dinner:** Large, fresh raw vegetable salad with *Dijon-Cider Dressing, Simple Detox Pizza*, steamed vegetables or *Hearty Vegetable Stew* as desired

**Dessert:** 3 Kollar cookies or ⅓ bar Dagoba 75-percent chocolate

## Day 6

**Upon rising:** A piece of fresh fruit

**Breakfast** (at least 20 minutes later): Sprouted grain toast with fresh avocado slices and 3 celery stalks

**Lunch:** *Italian Salad* with *Raw Caesar Dressing, Hearty Vegetable Stew*, 4 Ak-Mak crackers

**Snack** (at least 2 hours later): 1 to 2 glasses fresh carrot or mixed-vegetable juice, 1 bag of baby carrots and/or any raw vegetables of choice

**Dinner:** *Guacamole Salad, Detox Quesadilla*, steamed vegetables as desired

**Dessert:** 3 Kollar cookies or ⅓ bar Dagoba 75-percent chocolate

## Day 7

**Upon rising:** A piece of fresh fruit

**Breakfast** (at least 20 minutes later): Sprouted grain toast with fresh avocado slices and 3 celery stalks

**Lunch:** Large, fresh raw vegetable salad, *Liquid Gold Elixir* salad dressing, 1 avocado, *Raw Chocolate Pudding*

**Snack:** 1 bag of baby carrots and 4 Ak-Mak crakers

**Dinner:** Large, fresh raw vegetable salad, 2 sweet potatoes, 2 to 3 slices of sprouted grain toast (organic butter or raw honey optional), steamed vegetables as desired

**Dessert:** 3 Kollar cookies or ⅓ bar Dagoba 75-percent chocolate

# DETOX TRANSITION LEVEL 4

**Personal Profile** The typical Level 4 is approximately 45 to 35 pounds overweight. He or she has maintained a largely standard American diet, likely including lots of diet sodas and "low-quality" packaged, processed foods. This person may also be relatively thin but a junk food junkie, who is highly stressed and eats whatever can be obtained quickly and easily, possibly often on the road. This level is designed for those who have not made exercise and healthful eating a part of their regular lifestyle. Level 4's find themselves at fast food restaurants occasionally and battle cravings for sweets and starchy comfort foods.

## The Raw Food Detox Diet Menu for Level 4

(Italicized recipes are in this book)

### Day 1

**Breakfast:** Your favorite fresh fruit throughout the morning as desired (1 glass of raw fruit juice may be included, but it is advisable to dilute fresh apple or grape juice with water. Orange, grapefruit, and watermelon juice do not need to be diluted and are excellent choices as they are deeply hydrating.)

**Lunch:** *Ambrosia* with *Liquid Gold Elixir* salad dressing, Lara bar

**Snack** (3 to 4 hours later): Fresh fruit as desired

**Dinner:** *Classic Chopped Salad, Whole Wheat Lasagna*

**Dessert:** 3 Kollar cookies or ⅓ bar Dagoba 75-percent chocolate

**Day 2**

**Breakfast:** Your favorite fresh fruit throughout the morning as desired (1 glass of raw fruit juice may be included)

**Lunch:** *Raw Blended Carrot Renew*, raw flax seed crackers, raw vegetable salad with dressing of choice

**Snack:** (at least 3 hours later): Fresh fruit as desired

**Dinner:** *Italian Salad, Raw Caesar Dressing,* 1 bowl kamut pasta topped with steamed broccoli and Seeds of Change pasta sauce

**Dessert:** 3 Kollar cookies or *Hot Chocolate* and ⅓ bar Dagoba 75-percent chocolate

**Day 3**

**Breakfast:** Your favorite fresh fruit throughout the morning as desired (1 glass of raw fruit juice may be included)

**Lunch:** *Gazpacho,* raw flax seed crackers or raw granola bar, raw vegetable salad with dressing of choice

**Snack:** (at least 3 hours later): Fresh fruit as desired or 8 to 20 ounces *Green Lemonade*

**Dinner:** *Endive Bruschetta* and sliced raw vegetables of choice, *Maple-Glazed Salmon*, steamed vegetables as desired

**Dessert:** ⅓ bar Dagoba 75-percent chocolate or up to ⅓ package Alta Dena raw cheddar-style goat cheese

**Day 4**

**Breakfast:** Your favorite fresh fruit throughout the morning as desired (1 glass of raw fruit juice may be included)

**Lunch:** *Cranberry-Beet Medley Salad* with *Liquid Gold Elixir*, Lara bar or 4-ounce mix of your favorite raw nuts and dried fruits

**Snack** (3 to 4 hours later): Glass of fresh vegetable juice followed at least 20 minutes later by 1 bag of baby carrots and/or 1 small box of organic raisins

**Dinner:** Large, fresh raw vegetable salad (goat cheese optional), organic chicken (baked, rotisserie, or roasted), 1 to 2 cups steamed vegetables

**Dessert:** ⅓ bar Dagoba 75-percent chocolate

**Day 5**

**Breakfast:** Your favorite fresh fruit throughout the morning as desired (1 glass of raw fruit juice may be included)

**Lunch:** Large, fresh raw vegetable salad with *Liquid Gold Elixir* salad dressing and an *Avocado-Vegetable Sandwich*

**Predinner** (at least 20 minutes before your dinner meal): *Power Soup*

**Dinner:** *Classic Chopped Salad, Simple Detox Pizza* with steamed vegetables or *Hearty Vegetable Stew* as desired

**Dessert:** 3 Kollar cookies or ⅓ bar Dagoba 75-percent chocolate

## Day 6

**Breakfast:** Your favorite fresh fruit throughout the morning as desired (1 glass of raw fruit juice may be included)

**Lunch:** Raw vegetable salad and raw dressing of choice, sprouted grain bagel, 1 avocado, steamed vegetables as desired

**Snack:** (at least 2 hours later): 8 to 20 ounces *Green Lemonade*, 1 bag of baby carrots and/or any raw vegetables of choice

**Dinner:** *Fountain of Flavor Salad, Chilean Sea Bass with Creamy Port Sauce*

**Dessert:** ⅓ bar Dagoba 75-percent chocolate, up to ⅓ package Alta Dena raw cheddar-style goat cheese

## Day 7

**Breakfast:** Your favorite fresh fruit throughout the morning as desired (1 glass of raw fruit juice may be included)

**Lunch:** *Classic Chopped Salad with Dijon-Cider Dressing, Lentil-Curry Soup*, 4 Ak-Mak crackers

**Snack:** (at least 3 hours later): Fresh-squeezed orange juice, 2 bananas, or *Green Lemonade*

**Dinner:** *Classic Chopped Salad*, 2 sweet potatoes, 2 to 3 slices of sprouted grain toast (organic butter or raw honey optional), steamed vegetables as desired

**Dessert:** 3 Kollar cookies and 1 cup *Hot Chocolate*

# DETOX TRANSITION LEVEL 3

**Personal Profile** There's a range of typical Level 3's just coming into this lifestyle, but they all attempt to follow a healthful (and usually weight-loss specific) diet. The operative word here is "attempt." Sadly, Level 3's have fallen prey to common diet and health misconceptions. They avoid fresh fruits and carrots because they believe their calorie and sugar count will make them fat. They may tend toward soy products like tofu, soy chips, soy milk, and other widely misunderstood foods like peanut butter and protein shakes. They usually do not consume nearly enough fresh food. They may have started and stopped innumerable trend diets in attempts to get or stay at their desired weight. Many Level 3's are busy business-people or multitasking moms who try to make good choices but wind up giving in to convenience and temptation. Level 3's are usually under forty years old and do not have any major health issues.

## The Raw Food Detox Diet Menu for Level 3

(Italicized recipes are in this book)

### Day 1

**First thing in your stomach, whenever desired:** 8 to 20 ounces *Green Lemonade*

**Breakfast:** Your favorite fresh fruit throughout the morning as desired (1 glass of raw fruit juice may be included)

**Lunch:** *Classic Chopped Salad* with *Carrot-Ginger Dressing* and Lara bar

**Snack:** (3 to 4 hours later): Super Smoothie or *Green Lemonade*

**Dinner:** *Gazpacho* and *Maple-Glazed Salmon* with steamed vegetables

**Dessert:** ⅓ bar Dagoba 75-percent chocolate

### Day 2

**First thing in your stomach:** 8 to 20 ounces *Green Lemonade*

**Breakfast:** Your favorite fresh fruit throughout the morning as desired (1 glass of raw fruit juice may be included)

**Lunch:** *Raw Blended Carrot Renew*, large raw salad with sprouts and served with *Oh-So-Simple Romaine Wraps*

**Snack** (at least 3 hours later): *Sunshine Joy*, fresh fruit as desired or *Green Lemonade*

**Dinner:** *Classic Chopped Salad* with *Dijon-Cider Dressing*, 1 medium or large sweet potato, and 1 to 3 slices sprouted grain toast

**Dessert:** 3 Kollar cookies or *Hot Chocolate* and ⅓ bar Dagoba 75-percent chocolate

### Day 3

**First thing in your stomach:** 8 to 20 ounces *Green Lemonade*

**Breakfast:** Your favorite fresh fruit throughout the morning as desired (1 glass of raw fruit juice may be included)

**Lunch:** *Gazpacho,* raw flax seed crackers or raw granola bar, raw vegetable salad and dressing of choice

**Snack** (at least 3 hours later): Fresh fruit as desired or *Green Lemonade*

**Dinner:** *Raw Harvest Butternut and Coconut Soup, Fountain of Flavor Salad,* 3 slices sprouted grain toast (organic butter or raw honey optional)

**Dessert:** ⅓ bar Dagoba 75-percent chocolate or up to ⅓ package Alta Dena raw cheddar-style goat cheese

### Day 4

**First thing in your stomach:** 8 to 20 ounces *Green Lemonade*

**Breakfast:** Your favorite fresh fruit throughout the morning as desired (1 glass of raw fruit juice may be included)

**Lunch:** *Cranberry-Beet Medley Salad* with *Liquid Gold Elixir,* Lara bar or 4-ounce mix of your favorite raw nuts and dried fruits

**Snack** (3 to 4 hours later): *Green Lemonade* followed at least 20 minutes later by 1 bag of baby carrots and/or 1 small box of organic raisins

**Dinner:** Large raw vegetable salad topped with *Liquid Gold Elixir* and steamed vegetables with natural marinara sauce

**Dessert:** ⅓ bar Dagoba 75-percent chocolate

## Day 5

**First thing in your stomach:** 8 to 20 ounces *Green Lemonade*

**Breakfast:** Your favorite fresh fruit throughout the morning as desired (1 glass of raw fruit juice may be included)

**Lunch:** *Guacamole Salad, Raw Chocolate Pudding,* 2 young coconuts (save water for a beverage to enjoy whenever you like) or 2 bananas

**Predinner** (at least 20 minutes before your dinner meal): *Sunshine Joy* or *Power Soup*

**Dinner:** *Classic Chopped Salad, Sprouted-Grain Portobello Mushroom Fajitas*

**Dessert:** 3 Kollar cookies or ⅓ bar Dagoba 75-percent chocolate

## Day 6

**First thing in your stomach:** 8 to 20 ounces *Green Lemonade*

**Breakfast:** Your favorite fresh fruit throughout the morning as desired (1 glass of raw fruit juice may be included)

**Lunch:** Raw vegetable salad with raw dressing of choice, Lara bar or *Simple Pecan "Pie"* or 4 ounces of your favorite raw nuts and/or dried fruits

**Snack** (at least 2 hours later): 8 to 30 ounces *Green Lemonade* or 1 bag of baby carrots and/or any raw vegetables of choice

**Dinner:** *Raw Rainbow Salad* with *Liquid Gold Elixir* or *Carrot-Ginger Dressing, Chilean Sea Bass with Creamy Port Sauce,* steamed vegetables as desired

**Dessert:** ⅓ bar Dagoba 75-percent chocolate or up to ⅓ package Alta Dena raw cheddar-style goat cheese

## Day 7

**First thing in your stomach:** 8 to 20 ounces *Green Lemonade*

**Breakfast:** Your favorite fresh fruit throughout the morning as desired (1 glass of raw fruit juice may be included)

**Lunch:** *Classic Chopped Salad* with *Dijon-cider Dressing, Lentil-Curry Soup,* raw granola bar or raw flax seed crackers

**Snack** (at least 3 hours later): *Green Lemonade*

**Dinner:** *Classic Chopped Salad,* 2 sweet potatoes, 2 to 3 slices of sprouted grain toast, (organic butter or raw honey optional), steamed vegetables as desired

**Dessert:** 3 Kollar cookies and 1 cup *Hot Chocolate*

# DETOX TRANSITION LEVEL 2

**Personal Profile** A Level 2 has the motivation and desire to eat a mainly raw food diet but may also have the kind of lifestyle that demands that he or she frequently dine out. A Level 2 is not necessarily overweight but wants to get as lean as possible and obtain vibrant health. A Level 2 knows how to make good choices but realizes that by eating high-vibration foods and cleansing the colon, he or she can enjoy a whole new level of health. A Level 2 is not afraid of going the extra mile and is not overly attached to mainstream food. Since this is the second most demanding level of the Raw Food Detox Diet, it is not for everyone.

To be successful at Level 2, you must appreciate the kitchen and shop for fresh produce regularly. There are always ways around this, like having food delivered to your home by organic farms—such as Urban Organics in New York. Level 2's need to keep high-quality foods like raw nuts, dates, dried fruits, and raw treats around to help round out their raw meals. Do not venture to Level 2 unless you are really ready for it emotionally and physically. A good candidate for this level is a young person raised on natural foods or an athlete who has not used drugs or steroids and has not consumed large amounts of animal protein. If this does not describe you, you should spend some time at the previous levels before starting Level 2. Level 2's should also be willing to do some colon therapy if the need arises.

## A Note About Breakfast

At this level you do not consume fresh fruit until you have had your Green Lemonade or until noon. At this level you won't become light-headed or ravenous for lunch because your body is now used to taking very little in the morning. The aim is to keep your body clear (water is fine) until you actually feel the need for nourishment. This may be earlier on some days and later on others. One morning you may be ready for your Green Lemonade at 10:30 A.M. Another day you may not desire anything until 1:00 P.M. As long as you're not straining or forcing yourself to wait, you can wait as long as you feel comfortable before consuming your first fruit or vegetable juice of the day.

If you cannot get your vegetable juice before your fruit—or at all—on some days, don't worry. Just do your best to get it as often as possible (at least four to five days a week). If you miss a couple of days, try to double up on Green Lemonade the next day.

You may eat as much fruit as you like. It is best to stick to mono-fruit meals (one type of fruit at a time) at this level. If you like watermelon, feel free to eat as much as you want—I can easily put away half a watermelon at a sitting. If you're eating fruit until dinner, you might eat the whole melon. In the winter, grapefruits are wonderful and they mix perfectly with oranges. (You might eat 3 grapefruits and a couple of navel oranges followed by a couple of bananas. That's okay! It really is okay to eat as much as you like, as long as you're not mixing the fruit with any other food.)

As always, stop eating fruit at least *thirty minutes* before your afternoon meal to ensure that the fruit has a chance to exit the stomach before the next meal enters it.

## The Raw Food Detox Diet Menu for Level 2

(Italicized recipes are in this book)

### Day 1

**Mid-morning or when you first desire something:** *Green lemonade*

**Further along in the day:** Fresh fruit as desired

**Afternoon meal:** *Raw Rainbow Salad, Carrot-Ginger Dressing,* Lara bar

**Snack:** *Green Lemonade*

**Dinner:** *Power Soup, Raw Neutral Pasta Pesto,* 4 to 6 slices of Good Stuff raw bread (see appendix) with extra pesto

**Dessert:** *Raw Chocolate Ice Cream,* Blessing's Mega Raweo (see appendix)

### Day 2

**Mid-morning or when something is needed:** *Green Lemonade*

**Further along in the day:** Fresh fruit as desired

**Afternoon meal:** *Guacamole Salad* and *Raw Chocolate Pudding*

**Snack:** *Green Lemonade*

**Dinner:** *Thai Coconut Bliss, Cranberry-Beet Medley Salad*, raw crackers or Good Stuff raw bread.

**Dessert:** *Raw Chocolate Ice Cream*, raw bakery brownie

## Day 3

**Mid-morning or when something is needed:** *Green Lemonade*

**Further along in the day:** Fresh fruit as desired

**Afternoon meal:** Unlimited *Power Soup* followed at least 15 minutes later by a Lara bar

**Snack:** *Green Lemonade*

**Dinner:** *Raw Blended Carrot Renew, Simple Raw Sushi*

**Dessert:** Dee Dee's Sun Gems and/or a raw bakery brownie

## Day 4

**Mid-morning or when something is needed:** *Green Lemonade*

**Further along in the day:** Fresh fruit as desired

**Afternoon meal:** *Creamy Asian Salad* and Lara bar

**Snack:** *Green Lemonade*

**Dinner:** *Ambrosia Salad* and *Raw Neutral Pasta Pesto, Simple Pasta Marinara*, or *Kombi Pomodoro*, 4 to 6 slices Good Stuff raw bread with extra marinara

**Dessert:** *Hot Chocolate*, 3 to 4 small Raweos or one Mega Raweo (by Blessing's)

## Day 5

**Mid-morning or when something is needed:** *Green Lemonade*

**Further along in the day:** Fresh fruit as desired

**Afternoon meal:** *Classic Chopped Salad* topped with cranberries and pine nuts, if desired.

**Snack:** *Green Lemonade*

**Dinner:** *Kombu Pomodoro, Fresh Herb Cucumber Rolls*, Govinda Purple Power crackers or any raw crackers or Good Stuff bread.

**Dessert:** *Raw Cinnamon Apple-Pear Pie* or any raw treat desired

## Day 6

**Mid-morning or when something is needed:** *Green Lemonade*

**Further along in the day:** Fresh fruit as desired

**Afternoon meal:** *Oh-So-Simple-Romaine Wraps* and a bag of organic carrots

**Snack:** *Green Lemonade*

**Dinner:** *Power Soup, Raw Pad Thai*
**Dessert:** *Raw Strawberry Ice Cream*

## Day 7

**Mid-morning or when something is needed:** *Green Lemonade*
**Further along in the day:** Fresh fruit as desired
**Afternoon meal:** *Creamy Asian Salad*
**Snack:** *Green Lemonade*
**Predinner** (if desired): ⅓ package Alta Dena raw goat cheese or *Raw Goat Cheese Cabbage Sandwich*
**Dinner:** Grilled fish of your choice with steamed or lightly sautéed vegetables
**Dessert:** ⅓ bar Dagoba 75-percent chocolate or up to ⅓ package Alta Dena raw cheddar-style goat cheese

# DETOX TRANSITION LEVEL 1

**Personal Profile** A Level 1 has been through the other levels at some point before undertaking this level of the Raw Food Detox Diet. A Level 1 has probably spent sufficient time in the kitchen making raw foods fun and delicious. Otherwise he or she has extremely simple tastes and is easily satisfied with nature's unadulterated banquet. But a Level 1 could also be a gourmand who thoroughly enjoys food and the pleasures of the palate and is successfully marrying that aspect of themselves with the unrivaled pleasure of living in a clean, lean, vibrant body.

The meal payoffs for a Level 1 are large dinners and desserts. You can eat as much raw ice cream (if you use the recipe in this book) and as many raw treats as you desire.

Level 1's do not eat much during the day by choice. At this level, you learn that eating makes you less productive and less clear. Green juices and fruits are all you need and desire. If this way of eating doesn't feel right to you, it's not yet time for you to venture into Level 1 territory. You will know you're ready when it feels pleasurable—not like a form of hardship or deprivation.

To be successful at Level 1, it really helps to be creative with your raw dishes. Knowing how different raw flavors play off one another is critical because, even at this level, you still want your food to be full-flavored, ultra-pleasurable, comforting, and multitextured. The surest way to gain this kind of expertise is simply to practice by making lots of raw recipes like the ones coming up in part III of this book. Like Level 2's, you will be consuming a lot of raw produce, so find ways to make obtaining high-quality produce easy. Have standing orders for delivery. Keep your fridge well stocked with raw treats.

Do not venture to Level 1 unless you are really ready for it emotionally and physically. A good candidate for Level 1 is a person who feels great at Level 2 and, while extremely dedicated to this dieting style, is *not* overly obsessive about food. In other words, a Level 1 needs to be careful not to look at food as a religion and should absolutely be ready to do some colon therapy if symptoms (i.e., sluggishness, headaches, pimples, bouts of moodiness) pop up. It's a good idea for anyone wishing to reach Level 1 to spend at least one month at Level 2 first, unless they have been a raw foodist for awhile.

## A note about breakfast

At this level, fresh fruit is not typically consumed until you have had your Green Lemonade, which is not taken immediately upon rising, but rather after eleven or twelve o'clock. Often you won't desire fruit until later in the afternoon. For optimum clarity, some Level 1's don't consume anything but the juice until dinner a couple of times a week. This kind of "mini-fasting" allows the digestive system to clear any residual digestive matter, preventing even the smallest pile-up. Contrary to what you may be thinking, this leaves a Level 1 feeling highly energized. At this level, you will not become light-headed or be ravenous for lunch because your body has become used to taking in very little in the morning. And no, this does not slow down your metabolism! When your body is in a state of digestive rest, everything actually speeds up. Level 1's simply do not imbibe or ingest until they actually feel the need to do so—a novel concept, right? Like Level 2's, you can wait as long as you feel comfortable (without straining or forcing yourself) before consuming your first fruit or vegetable juice of the day.

If you cannot get your vegetable juice before your fruit—or at all—on some days, just do your best to get it as often as possible (at least four to five days a week). If you miss a couple of days, try to double up on Green Lemonade the next day, or just let it go. It's up to you.

## The Raw Food Detox Diet Menu for Level 1

(Italicized recipes are in this book)

### Day 1
**Noon:** *Green Lemonade*
**Throughout the day:** Fresh fruit as desired
**Snack:** *Green Lemonade* and/or more fruit
**Dinner:** *Power Soup, Rawviolis,* raw bread with extra raw marinara
**Dessert:** *Raw Strawberry Ice Cream* and 1 young coconut

### Day 2
**Noon:** *Green Lemonade*
**Throughout the day:** Fresh fruit as desired
**Snack:** *Green Lemonade*

**Dinner:** *Thai Coconut Bliss, Raw Pad Thai*

**Dessert** Raw brownie and/or raw pecan pie bar

## Day 3

**Noon:** *Green Lemonade*

**Throughout the day:** Fresh fruit as desired

**Snack:** *Green Lemonade*

**Dinner:** *Raw Blended Carrot Renew, Guacamole Salad*

**Dessert:** 1 to 2 young coconuts, 1 cup *Raw Chocolate Pudding*

## Day 4

**Noon:** *Green Lemonade*

**Throughout the day:** Fresh fruit as desired

**Snack:** *Green Lemonade*

**Dinner:** *Creamy Asian Salad* with sliced almonds, *Oh-So-Simple Romaine Wraps*

**Dessert:** Your favorite *Raw Ice Cream* and ⅓ bar Dagoba 75-percent chocolate

## Day 5

**Noon:** *Green Lemonade*

**Throughout the day:** Fresh fruit as desired

**Dinner:** *Simple Raw Sushi, Arame Salad* and *Japanese "Rice"*

**Dessert:** Your favorite *Raw Ice Cream*

## Day 6

**Noon:** *Green Lemonade*

**Throughout the day:** Fresh fruit as desired

**Snack:** *Green Lemonade*

**Dinner:** *Ambrosia,* raw bread with *Raw Neutral Pasta Pesto*

**Dessert:** *Raw Cinnamon Apple-Pear Pie* with *Raw Vanilla Ice Cream*

## Day 7

**Noon:** *Green Lemonade*

**Throughout the Day:** Fresh fruit as desired

**Snack:** *Green Lemonade*

**Pre-Dinner:** 1 to 2 pounds organic carrots

**Dinner:** Raw green salad, steamed vegetables with marinara sauce, and *Maple-Glazed Salmon* or other grilled fish

**Dessert:** ⅓ bar Dagoba 75-percent chocolate

# MY EXPERIENCE AS A LEVEL 1

Almost every client in the history of my practice has asked me what I eat in a day. The other most popular question is, "Does your husband eat this way, too?" Given their curiosity, I can only guess that you are wondering the same thing.

I am a Level 1, but I spent many years at Levels 5, 4, 3, and 2 to get here. I spent about two years at Level 5. From there I moved rapidly through Level 3 where I experienced the most dramatic weight loss. I found Level 3 very easy because I could look forward to a cooked meal every night if I so desired. I loved Level 3 because I loved comfort foods and starches like the sweet potatoes, sprouted grain breads, and whole grain cookies. This was the point at which I developed and grew my practice. As my body cleansed more deeply, I leaped to Level 2 where I grew more comfortable going days at a time on an all-raw meal plan. And then, one day about four years ago, I found myself surprisingly content at Level 1.

If you had told me ten years ago that I would one day live on a nearly all-raw plant food diet, I wouldn't have believed it. I was heavily addicted to stimulating foods, particularly bagels and frozen yogurt. But the gentle transition made it really easy. Moreover, after years of struggling with my weight, the results made the effort so worthwhile!

I practice what I preach in my family life as well. I have followed this dieting program through two pregnancies and while nursing my babies. Both times, I was able to recover my ideal shape in record time and without stress.

As for my husband and children, they are fully content to eat this way—but I am never strict with them and would never keep them from enjoying a food that I wouldn't recommend. I also loosen the reins on my kids when they go to parties or when we travel. It's important for children to feel like they can make their own choices, and usually the amount of low-quality foods they consume on such an occasion is minimal anyway. I know that once they are home again it's back to the good stuff!

Without focusing on it, my husband eats many all-raw meals each week, and aside from the occasional birthday party, my kids only eat natural, mostly raw foods. Both of my kids can suck down a glass of Green Lemonade and have even been known to fight for the last sip!

## My typical day looks something like this:

**Around noon:** 30 ounces Green Lemonade

**1 to 5 P.M.:** A whole watermelon or other abundant fresh fruit

**6:30 P.M.:** Predinner nosh on cherry tomatoes and organic carrots
(occasionally with a glass of wine)

**7:30 P.M.:** Large gourmet raw salad or raw entrée/soup, all the raw

bread or other savory raw treats I desire (for example, a loaf of
raw bread layered with fresh pesto, raw honey, or made into an
open-face sandwich with sliced tomatoes, alfalfa, and Dijon
mustard), 1 bowl raw ice cream, raw brownie and/or other sweet
raw treat, and possibly a glass of wine.

If I am eating an occasional cooked meal, it will probably consist of steamed veggies with marinara sauace and/or a couple of sweet potatoes with a hearty avocado salad, and dark chocolate for
dessert. Occasionally, at one of my favorite New York City restaurants, I will have a piece of fish
with veggies. I'll always start with a green salad (possibly with goat cheese) or, in summer, a bowl
of Gazpacho. When eating out, I'll always enjoy a glass or two of wine. Then I'll save dessert for
when I come home, where my favorite dark chocolate is always waiting. Sometimes, if I'm feeling "peckish," I'll slice up some Alta Dena raw cheddar-style goat cheese as well.

You see, while I am strict about some things like almost always having my green juice,
never eating in the morning, only eating raw fruits (or sometimes greens) before dinner, and always eating quick exit combinations, I am very liberal about following my cravings. I eat as much
as I desire and make sure there are safe ways for me to indulge—that's where chocolate, raw goat
cheese, great meals out, and good wine come in! These are the tricks to getting everything you
want.

I probably eat much more "calorically" speaking than I did when I weighed 30 pounds
more. It goes to show that calories are not the issue. Quick exit foods that the body can recognize
(at the right times, and in quick exit combinations) put low-calorie "diet" foods to shame any day
of the week! I have not counted a calorie or fat gram for years; I enjoy hearty, unmeasured portions of my favorite quick exit foods; and I'm leaner than I ever imagined possible—even after
giving birth to two children.

It bears repeating that I could never have conceived of eating this way in my past food-life.
Dense, cooked foods were too much a part of my lifestyle to have believed that I could be satisfied or content eating at this raw food level. I would have thought it sheer deprivation. But that's
how it seems before your cells get cleaned. Now, the very thought of eating the way I used to
seems like torture. So don't be too quick to look at Level 1 and think, "I could never do that. If
that's what this is all about, it's not for me." Level 1 may or may not be for you. But Levels 4 and
5 are for everyone, and for many of you, that is enough to get you feeling and looking better than
you ever dreamed possible!

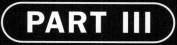

**PART III**

# THE RAW FOOD DETOX DIET RECIPES

# RAW FOOD DETOX RECIPE LIST

# HOW TO USE
# THESE RECIPES

The recipes are laid out in three sections: *The Fundamentals* are the key recipes for the program that everyone should make. This section includes Liquid Gold Elixir, the heavenly elixir salad dressing that has garnered worldwide acclaim from publications ranging from *Daily Candy Everywhere* to *Elle Italia*. This dressing is a "must make," as it will make your salads come alive with flavor, you may use it liberally, and it lasts up to two weeks in the fridge! While you can still have great success on the Raw Food Detox Diet without making *The Fundamentals*, you will see the best results and effect better internal healing in the long run if you incorporate them into the program.

The second section, *Expanding Your Repertoire*, offers additional basic (but in no way boring), weight-loss-inducing, beautifying recipes. This more expansive recipe section is home to healthier versions of your favorite dishes, sauces, and desserts—all with simplicity in mind.

For the adventurous gourmand, there is the third recipe section, *Masterful Creations*—this is for the reader who likes to spend time in the kitchen and is easily inspired by new ingredients and flavors. While these recipes are not difficult, they do require a touch of artistry by breaking away from the predictable. Readers who are drawn to this section will probably thrive at transition Level 1 or 2; mastering these recipes will ensure that they will never tire of their raw meals, particularly when eating raw for dinner. Many of these recipes are highly simplified renditions of gourmet dishes, without losing any of the core pleasure of the dish—a very special section indeed!

Finally, I've included an entertainer's section for dinner parties, *Sample Menus For Entertaining*, so that you can easily weave this aspect of your lifestyle into your social events and show your friends how indulgent eating this way can be!

Next to each of the recipes, you will see numbers listed. Each number represents the transition level (1 to 5) for which the recipe is designed. If you see a "D" next to the transition level, you'll know that the dish is ideally meant for dinner at that level. Also note that, while your particular level may not be listed next to a dish, you can always make room for that dish on occasion. For example, a Level 1 will not typically have the Whole Wheat Lasagna, but that doesn't mean a Level 1 can never have it—just that it is not a staple of a Level 1 program. There is a time and place for every recipe, no matter what your level.

While I have included approximate serving sizes, keep in mind that you may enjoy unlimited amounts of any dishes made purely from raw vegetables or fresh fruits, such as the raw vegetable salads and raw soups. If the recipe calls for concentrated or cooked ingredients, be careful not to eat more than a satisfying helping of that dish.

Please also note that none of these recipes call for dehydration, soaking, or sprouting. This is to underscore the fact that these processes are unnecessary in the Raw Food Detox Diet. These dishes are all created with your busy schedule in mind. They also require minimal kitchen appliances. You should have a good set of knives, a solid wooden chopping block, and I highly recommend purchasing a K-Tec Champ HP Blender (see page 99). This is the best blender on the market, and it comes in handy when preparing a lot of raw soups—and particularly the raw ice creams, which require blending ice effortlessly. However, you will find plenty of recipes here that do not require any special equipment.

There is only minimal use of raw fats in these recipes. While raw fats are good and important on many levels, most raw food recipes call for too much plant-based fat. Even the best fats should be used carefully, as they are very dense and difficult to break down. This is especially true for women, who have a hard time breaking down fats in general. Women should also be especially careful of raw recipes and raw restaurants that use large amounts of coconut butter. On that note, be sure to store your fats properly. Raw nuts should be kept refrigerated. Olive oil should be purchased in dark glass containers, kept cool, and stored away from the light (keeping a pantry away from the oven is usually a good bet). Avocados should never be too soft, as this means the fat content is probably rancid—and rancid fats, in addition to being difficult to digest, can give you a debilitating headache and/or stomachache.

Seasoned chefs and novices alike will be able to make every one of these detox recipes. The only difference between the two levels of chefs vis-à-vis the recipes will be *confidence*. Confidence is an essential ingredient. Enthusiasm and passion must also be infused into every recipe here, or in any other book, for that matter. These are your Raw Food Detox Diet recipe mantras:

■ Absolutely, I can make this!

■ I love making these healthy dishes!

■ I am nourishing my body and soul with healing food for a beautiful, joyful life!

In preparing cleansing food, you will in no way sacrifice flavor. You will still enjoy the basic tastes that every well-balanced palate desires: sweet, salty, fatty, acidic/sour, and spicy. Here are everyday ingredients that I recommend you keep handy in your kitchen to facilitate the preparation of your favorite detox dishes:

**For sweetness:**
100 percent pure maple syrup
New White Stevia
Raw honey
Dates
Dried fruit
Agave nectar

**For saltiness:**
Nama Shoyu (raw soy sauce)
Celtic sea salt
Seaweed

**For fattiness:**
Raw nuts
Cold-pressed oils
Avocados
Young coconuts

**For acidity/sourness:**
Fresh citrus juice
Various vinegars (in small quantities) such as balsamic, white wine,
        sherry, and so forth.

**For spice:**
Fresh herbs
Curries
Fresh ginger
Garlic

In addition to making sure your dishes meet all of your palate's desires, I encourage you to use the freshest, organic produce you can find (when you can get it). Also, whenever possible, use fresh herbs, garlic, and ginger. The dried and powdered versions will not give these dishes the desired boldness of flavor.

# ESSENTIAL DETOX APPLIANCES

(All of the following appliances can be found at www.highvibe.com/raw.)

**The Breville Fountain Juicer (or any other juicer of your choice that juices green, leafy vegetables easily)** I love the Breville because it's easy to use and clean, has a very large mouth, which means you don't have to cut up things like apples and lemons, and, at about $150, it's well priced.

**Mandolin** A mandolin is a kitchen appliance which allows you to slice vegetables very thin. This is my most frequently used food prep item as it enables me to turn vegetables into gourmet delicacies. After slicing vegetables into thin layers, I like to stack them and then slice again, creating matchstick pieces or even something akin to noodles. I also love to run beets over the mandolin to use as "rose petals" around the plate! You can buy one for about $30.

**Spiralizer** A spiralizer is an essential item for pasta fans. You can make pasta out of zucchini, carrots, squash, pumpkin, and much more by using this nifty contraption. It retails for about $25.

**The K-Tec Champ HP Blender** All I can say about this particular blender is that I use it at least three times every day. It will make your detox transition infinitely more enjoyable. Many people ask me why they need this if they already have a blender. You don't really need it unless you want to make any of the ice creams. But once you buy it, you will see how great it is to have on hand for *all* recipes that require blending. I use it to make fruit shakes, dressings, soups, and smoothies throughout the day. And I use it at least two or three times a week to make fresh, raw ice cream (my family and friends go through a lot of it very quickly!). While not inexpensive at $350, it is worth every penny (and comes with an eight-year warranty).

## HOW TO OPEN A YOUNG COCONUT

I used to be incredibly intimidated by young coconuts. In fact, I used to avoid every recipe calling for young coconuts because I thought they were impossible to find, let alone open. When I finally made the effort to find a place that carried them and purchased a cleaver, I started to use them all the time—in dishes, on their own, and for their water, which has become my children's favorite household drink.

Choose a preshaved, young coconut with a white exterior. Set the coconut on a firm, steady surface. I like to put it on a wooden chopping block as well, to protect my kitchen counter from nicks. Place your non-cleaver hand behind your back and leave it there no matter what happens—to ensure you don't lose it! Place the cleaver on the upper third of the coconut (about 4 inches from the peak of the coconut, and mark where you will strike it. Lift the cleaver to about shoulder height and, keeping your eye on the mark, come down on it with force. Work your way around the peak of the coconut such that, once you've made four or five cleaver marks, the top of the coconut will lift off like a little hat. Inside, it should look crisp and white. Enjoy the water or set it aside for later use, and then use a spoon to enjoy the coconut "flesh." Some coconuts will have firmer flesh than others.

# THE FUNDAMENTALS

## Green Lemonade (All Levels)

*I already provided this recipe and extolled its merits at great length in part I, but it is such an essential part of the Raw Food Detox Diet that I'm including it again here.*

**MAKES 1 SERVING**

**1 head romaine lettuce or celery**

**5 to 6 stalks kale (any type)**

**1 to 2 apples (as needed for sweetness—I recommend organic Fuji)**

**1 whole organic lemon (you don't have to peel it)**

**1 to 2 tablespoons fresh ginger (optional)**

Process the vegetables through the juicer by admitting one vegetable at a time through the mouth of the juicer. The fiber will shoot out of the juicer into one container while the spout will eject the fresh juice into another container. Pour into a large glass and drink! Notice how the lemon really cuts out the "green" taste that most people try to avoid.

# Liquid Gold Elixir (All Levels)

*When made correctly, this amazing dressing is the color of gold!*

**MAKES 4 CUPS**

2 cups fresh lemon juice
3 whole cloves garlic
3 tablespoon minced ginger
3 tablespoons Nama Shoyu soy sauce
3 heaping tablespoons raw honey (or more if desired)
1½ cups cold-pressed olive oil

Place all of the ingredients except the oil in blender. Begin blending at normal speed. As the mixture is blending, slowly add the oil until it's completely blended. This recipe should last over a week in the fridge.

# Sunshine Joy and Power Soup (All Levels)

*Both of these raw soups should be enjoyed ten to fifteen minutes before a meal or as a snack—always on an empty stomach. You can even enjoy them for breakfast. Chock-full of enzymes and water-containing fruits and vegetables, both soups are ideal for weight loss!*

## SUNSHINE JOY

**MAKES 2 TO 3 SERVINGS**

1 cup organic alfalfa sprouts

6 organic dates

2 cups fresh pineapple

3 leaves fresh kale,
   removed from stem

1–2 tablespoons packed fresh mint

## POWER SOUP

**MAKES 2 TO 3 SERVINGS**

1 cup organic alfalfa sprouts

3 cups fresh strawberries

3 tablespoons raw honey

2–4 packets Stevia
   (if desired for extra sweetness)

1 large head Romaine lettuce

$\frac{1}{4}$ medium beet (optional for a
   deep red color for the soup)

Blend until very smooth. You may want to blend in a couple of ice cubes as well so that the mixture does not heat up while blending. The soup is best when served immediately, but it will last in the refrigerator for 2 days.

# EXPANDING YOUR REPERTOIRE

*These recipes are simple and delicious. These flavorful dishes are created using fresh herbs and savvy slicing—no complicated dehydration or other time-consuming measures!*

## Soups

### Hearty Vegetable Stew

(LEVELS 1D, 2D, 3D, 4, AND 5)

**MAKES 4 SERVINGS**

8 large carrots, chopped

5 stalks celery, chopped

1 leek, chopped

1 head broccoli, chopped

1 zucchini, chopped

1 cup chopped mushrooms

1 cup okra

$1/2$ medium onion

Equal parts water and Pacific vegetable broth to cover vegetables (about 6 cups)

**½ serrano chili (optional)**
**Spike to taste**
**Curry powder to taste**
**Celtic sea salt to taste**

Place the carrots, celery, leek, broccoli, zucchini, mushrooms, okra, onion (and any other vegetables you desire) into a large pot with the water, broth, chili, and spices. Bring the mixture to a boil and simmer until the carrots are semisoft. Best served with hot, sprouted grain toast with organic butter and/or raw honey.

As with all homemade soups, the longer the vegetables soak in the water (even while in the refrigerator), the more flavorful the soup will become. For a thicker soup, you may blend half the mixture then add it back to the batch.

# Lentil-Curry Soup

## (LEVELS 3D, 4, AND 5)

**MAKES 4 SERVINGS**

**Same vegetables as Hearty Vegetable Stew (page 104)**
**1½ cups black, brown, red, or green lentils**
**3 teaspoons curry powder (or more to taste)**
**1 bunch cilantro, chopped (optional) or 4 whole bay leaves chopped (optional)**

Boil the vegetables, lentils, and curry powder in a large pot and simmer until the lentils and carrots are cooked through (about 45 minutes). Top with the cilantro or bay leaves, if desired.

# Carrot–Sweet Potato Bisque

## (LEVELS 1D, 2D, 3D, 4, AND 5)

**MAKES 4 SERVINGS**

**2 sweet potatoes**

**2 cups baby carrots**

**1 cup water**

**2 cups Pacific vegetable broth**

**$\frac{1}{2}$ teaspoon Celtic sea salt**

**1 packet Splenda**

**$\frac{1}{4}$ teaspoon cumin**

**$\frac{1}{2}$ teaspoon coriander powder**

**$\frac{1}{4}$ teaspoon minced ginger**

**$\frac{1}{4}$ teaspoon minced garlic**

This soup is so easy (no chopping required). Bake the sweet potatoes and boil the carrots until soft. In a blender, mix all ingredients and process until uniform. Pour mixture into large saucepan and heat to taste.

# Raw Harvest Butternut and Coconut Soup (All Levels)

**MAKES 4 SERVINGS**

Meat of 2 young coconuts

1½ cups coconut water

1 cup butternut or pumpkin cubes (about 1-inch cubes)

8 organic dates or ⅓ cup pure maple syrup

1 pinch nutmeg, cinnamon, or pumpkin pie spice

Combine all the ingredients in a blender and blend on high until smooth. Enjoy!

# Raw Blended Carrot Renew (All Levels)

**MAKES 4 SERVINGS**

2 cups fresh carrot juice

1 ripe avocado

1 tablespoon curry powder

1 tablespoon fresh ginger

1 clove garlic

Blend all of the ingredients in a blender on high until smooth.

# Raw Curry Cantaloupe Soup (All Levels)

**MAKES 4 SERVINGS**

1 cantaloupe
½ teaspoon cinnamon
½ teaspoon nutmeg
½ teaspoon garam masala
½ teaspoon curry powder

Combine all ingredients in a blender and blend until smooth. Serve well-chilled in a bowl or a chilled cantaloupe half. Eat as much as you like!

# Gazpacho (All Levels)

**MAKES 4 SERVINGS**

**FOR THE SOUP BASE**

6 medium vine-ripe tomatoes, halved
½ to 1 cup packed fresh basil
⅓ cup apple cider vinegar
2 tablespoons olive oil
1 teaspoon Nama Shoyu soy sauce
1 clove garlic
1 to 2 teaspoons Spike
Celtic sea salt and freshly ground
      black pepper to taste

**FOR THE "MEAT"**

1 yellow bell pepper, finely chopped
1 to 2 cobs corn, kernels cut off the cob
½ apple, chopped
¼ jicama, chopped

**To make the base:** In a blender, combine all of the ingredients and blend until desired consistency is reached. You may use the whole tomatoes, including skin and seeds.

**To make the "meat":** Combine the chopped vegetables and fruit in a large bowl. Pour the base mixture into the bowl and mix well. Serve well-chilled. It tastes even better the next day!

# David Burke & Donatella's Classic Gazpacho (All Levels)

*David Burke & Donatella (at 133 East 61st Street) is possibly the best thing to appear on the New York City restaurant scene in recent years. The dynamic-duo restaurateurs behind the highly-acclaimed venue contributed this succulent raw soup recipe for use in this book. If you are fortunate enough to get a much-coveted reservation at their restaurant, you will find many detox-approved dishes on their menu, such as their Market Salad with fresh herbs, salmon, and dover sole. Order any of these with a side of vegetables and a glass of your favorite wine and enjoy!*

**MAKES 4 SERVINGS**

**5 large tomatoes, quartered**
**1/2 cucumber, peeled, seeded, and chopped**
**1/2 red bell pepper, chopped**
**2 cloves garlic**
**2 tablespoons coarse or kosher salt**
**1 teaspoon cayenne pepper**
**1/2 cup olive oil**

Place all the ingredients in a food processor and blend until finely puréed. Depending on the size of your processor, you may have to do this in two or more steps.

# Thai Carrot Soup

## (LEVELS 1D, 2D, 3, 4, AND 5)

**MAKES 4 SERVINGS**

15 carrots, cut into 1 to 2-inch slices

32 ounces Pacific vegetable broth

2 tablespoons lemon grass

1 small Spanish onion, chopped

3 tablespoons curry (or to taste)

3 tablespoons Spike

1 tablespoon minced ginger

2 to 3 cloves garlic

Fresh cilantro

Place the carrots, broth, lemon grass, and onion into a soup pot. Bring to a boil and simmer until the carrots are medium-soft (you should be able to pierce with a fork). Let it cool. Put small batches (about 2 cups at a time) of the mixture into your blender and purée. Once it's all puréed, add the curry, Spike, ginger, and garlic until it suits your taste. Serve with fresh cilantro.

# Dressings and Sauces

## Raw Tahini Dressing (All Levels)

**MAKES ABOUT 4 CUPS**

1 cup raw tahini

1/4 teaspoon cumin

1/2 teaspoon coriander

3 tablespoons apple juice concentrate

1 clove garlic

2 tablespoons Nama Shoyu soy sauce

1 tablespoon lemon juice

1 Splenda or stevia packet (if more sweetness is desired)

1/2 cup water or 1/3 cup apple cider vinegar

Blend all ingredients except water in a blender until smooth. This mixture thickens in the refrigerator. Add the water to dilute before serving.

## Dijon-Cider Dressing (All Levels)

**MAKES 1/2 CUP**

1 1/2 tablespoons Dijon mustard

1/3 cup apple cider vinegar

4 tablespoons cold-pressed olive oil

2 packets Splenda or stevia

Freshly ground pepper to taste

Blend all ingredients in a blender until smooth.

Keeps for 3 weeks.

# Raw Caesar Dressing (All Levels)

**MAKES 3 CUPS**

**¼ cup cold-pressed olive oil**
**2 cloves garlic, chopped**
**4 medium stalks celery, cut into thirds**
**½ cup water**
**¼ cup freshly squeezed lemon juice**
**¼ cup Nama Shoyu soy sauce**
**2 tablespoons sweet white miso**
**5 organic unsulfured dates**
**Freshly ground pepper to taste**

Blend all of the ingredients in blender and serve over romaine lettuce. This is a neutral dressing and may also be used as mayonnaise (use less water for a thicker consistency).

Keeps for about 10 days.

# Asian Dressing (All levels)

**MAKES ½ CUP**

2 tablespoons raw tahini

1 clove garlic, chopped

1 inch fresh ginger, chopped

1 lemon, juiced

2 to 3 packets stevia or Splenda or 2 tablespoons raw honey

1 teaspoon sesame oil

3 tablespoon Nama Shoyu soy sauce

Mix the ingredients in a bowl. I love this mixture over baby romaine, mung bean sprouts, and baby bok choy with chopped basil and cilantro.

Keeps for about 10 days.

# Raw Ranch Dressing (All Levels)

**MAKES 2 CUPS**

½ cup fresh lemon juice

1 tablespoon Celtic sea salt

1 tablespoon dried chives

1 tablespoon dried rosemary

1 tablespoon dried oregano

1 tablespoon dried sage

1 cup whole, raw macadamia nuts

⅓ cup cold-pressed olive oil (optional)

Blend all of the ingredients until very smooth. Add water to achieve desired consistency.

Keeps for 1 week.

# Carrot-Ginger Dressing (All Levels)

**MAKES 4 CUPS**

2½ cups baby carrots

3 tablespoons fresh ginger

4 to 5 packets Splenda or stevia

⅓ cup apple cider vinegar

½ cup water

1 clove garlic

¼ cup flax seed oil

1 drizzle sesame oil (as desired)

Cumin, coriander, or curry spice to taste

Blend all of the ingredients (using only ½ of the carrots) except the spice in a blender. Add the cumin, coriander, or curry to taste. As the mixture is blending, slowly add the additional carrots. You may need to add more water or apple cider vinegar to facilitate blending action. Use on salads or as a dip for raw sushi rolls or crudite.

Keeps for 2 weeks.

# Spring-in-Your-Step Rolls and Raw Teriyaki Sauce (All Levels)

**MAKES 10 SERVINGS**

**FOR THE TERIYAKI SAUCE**

1 cup Nama Shoyu soy sauce

1 cup pure maple syrup

1 teaspoon ginger, whole or chopped

1 clove garlic

1 drizzle toasted sesame oil

**FOR THE SPRING ROLLS**

1 red bell pepper, julienned

2 large carrots, julienned

1 bunch whole cilantro leaves

1 bunch mint leaves, chopped

1 bunch whole basil leaves

10 whole red or green cabbage leaves

**To make the sauce:** Blend all the ingredients and use as a dipping sauce for spring rolls, raw salad rolls, or rice paper rolls.

**To make the rolls:** Place the bell pepper, carrots, cilantro, mint, and basil inside a cabbage leaf. Roll the cabbage leaf and dip into the teriyaki sauce.

# Amazing Raw "Peanut" Sauce (All Levels)

*This tastes like an authentic Thai peanut sauce without using any peanuts.*

**MAKES 2 CUPS**

1 cup raw almond butter

2 tablespoons fresh ginger, whole or chopped

½ cup water (to thin)

4 tablespoon fresh lemon juice

¼ cup pure maple syrup

3 tablespoons Nama Shoyu soy sauce

4 teaspoon sesame oil

2 to 3 cloves garlic

½ serrano or jalapeño chile

Blend all ingredients at high speed until smooth. This makes an unbelievable dipping sauce for carrots or other vegetables, and it tastes amazing as a salad dressing or a sauce over young coconut noodles!

# Middle Eastern Nut Cheese (All Levels)

**MAKES ½ CUP**

**3 tablespoons pine nuts**

**3 tablespoons chopped macadamia nuts**

**3 tablespoons chopped walnuts**

**Juice of 1½ lemons**

**⅓ cup fresh parsley, chopped (add more if desired)**

**1 clove garlic**

**7 dashes Bragg's Liquid Aminos**

**Dash of Nama Shoyu soy sauce**

Blend all of the above ingredients in a blender until smooth. Use as a spread on vegetables or in raw sushi.

# Raw Salads and Other Raw Delights

## Creamy Asian Salad and Dressing (All Levels)

*This is one of the most delicious salads I have ever enjoyed!*

**MAKES 4 TO 6 SERVINGS**

**FOR THE SALAD**

2 cups mung bean sprouts

2 cups shredded green or
    purple cabbage

1 red bell pepper, thinly sliced

1 cup sugar snap peas

½ cup mushrooms (shiitake or
    button)

½ cup watercress, chopped

¼ cup fresh cilantro, chopped

2 tablespoons fresh basil, chopped

1 clove garlic, chopped

**FOR THE DRESSING**

1 inch ginger, chopped

1 cup cold-pressed olive oil

2 teaspoons toasted sesame oil

2 cloves garlic

2 tablespoons fresh minced ginger

4 tablespoons lemon juice

4 tablespoons sweet white miso

6 whole dates, pitted

2 tablespoons Nama Shoyu soy sauce

¼ cup water

**To make the salad:** Mix all of the ingredients together in a salad bowl. Set aside.

**To make the dressing:** Blend all ingredients in a blender until smooth. One hour before serving, pour half of the dressing over the salad. Mix thoroughly and enjoy!

# Oh-So-Simple Romaine Wraps (All Levels)

**MAKES 5 SERVINGS**

5 large romaine lettuce leaves
5 tablespoons raw almond butter
5 teaspoons raw honey

Spread 1 tablespoon of the almond butter and 1 teaspoon of the raw honey on each romaine leaf. Roll the romaine leaf and devour!

# Easy Raw Coleslaw (All Levels)

**MAKES 4 TO 6 SERVINGS**

1 cup shredded green cabbage
1 cup shredded red cabbage
¼ cup raisins
½ cup Liquid Gold Elixir (page 102)

Marinate the cabbage and the raisins in Liquid Gold Elixir for at least 1 hour before serving.

# Apple-Raisin Dream (All Levels)

**MAKES 4 SERVINGS**

¼ to ½ pound baby romaine lettuce

1 cup grape tomatoes, sliced in half

½ cup raisins

1 Fuji apple (or other crisp apple), finely chopped

3 tablespoons scallions, chopped

2 tablespoons chives, chopped

1 yellow or orange bell pepper, chopped

½ English cucumber, chopped

¼ cup packed fresh basil

Mix all of the ingredients in a salad bowl. Toss and serve with Liquid Gold Elixir (page 102).

# Hearty Corn Salad (All Levels)

*"Hearty" is the operative word. This salad makes you feel like you're eating a stew, but it digests absolutely seamlessly!*

**MAKES 4 SERVINGS**

**3 portobello mushrooms, chopped**

**1/3 cup balsamic vinegar**

**1/3 cup olive oil**

**3 tablespoons pure maple syrup**

**2 tablespoons sliced scallions**

**1 bell pepper (any color), chopped**

**1 cup grape tomatoes, sliced in half**

**1/4 to 1/2 pound baby lettuce**

**4 ears fresh corn, kernels cut from cob**

Marinate the mushrooms for 1 hour in the vinegar, olive oil, and maple syrup. Set aside.

Mix scallions, bell pepper, tomatoes, lettuce, and corn in a large bowl. Toss well. Divide lettuce mixture onto plates and top with 2 to 3 heaping tablespoons of the mushrooms. Dress salad further, if desired, with Raw Caesar Dressing (page 112).

# Classic Chopped Salad (All Levels)

**MAKES 4 SERVINGS**

1 cup fresh haricots verts (green beens)

3 ears fresh corn, kernels cut from cob

1 yellow bell pepper, chopped

2 large carrots, chopped

2 cups grape tomatoes, sliced in half

1 zucchini, chopped

3 tablespoons fresh chives, minced

Mix all ingredients in a large bowl.

# Ambrosia (All Levels)

*This dish is often served as the first course at my dinner parties. It really wakes up and pleases the palate!*

**MAKES 4 TO 6 SERVINGS**

**1 bell pepper, thinly sliced**

**1 large carrot, sliced into matchstick pieces**

**1 zucchini, sliced into matchstick pieces or thinly sliced with a carrot peeler**

**1 large beet, cut into matchstick pieces**

**½ cup chopped walnuts**

**1 cup apples, sliced into matchstick pieces**

**2 tablespoons fresh ginger, diced**

**2 cloves garlic, diced**

**½ jalapeño or serrano chili, diced**

**½ cup dried unsulfured cranberries**

**½ cup sliced sunchokes (Jerusalem artichokes; matchstick pieces)**

**¼ cup packed fresh mint**

**½ cup packed fresh basil**

**½ bunch packed fresh cilantro**

Mix all ingredients in a large bowl. Toss well and serve topped with Liquid Gold Elixir (page 102).

# Fountain of Flavor Salad (All Levels)

*Clove and cinnamon add wonderful elements of surprise to a dish. This salad warms your senses and triggers further creativity in the kitchen by mixing warm and tangy with a touch of Indian spice.*

**MAKES 4 SERVINGS**

1 cup cherry tomatoes, sliced in half

1 teaspoon cinnamon

1 teaspoon ground cloves

1 clove garlic, chopped

3 cups romaine lettuce, chopped

1$^1$/$_2$ teaspoons fresh oregano, chopped

1$^1$/$_2$ teaspoons fresh thyme, chopped

$^1$/$_4$ cup cold-pressed olive oil

2 tablespoons red wine vinegar

4 raw olives, chopped

Celtic sea salt and freshly ground pepper to taste

Add all of the ingredients into a mixing bowl. Toss well and enjoy! This is a neutral dish, so you can combine it with anything.

# Raw Rainbow Salad (All Levels)

*This is a simply beautiful creation that will appeal to everyone.*

**MAKES 2 TO 4 SERVINGS**

$\frac{1}{2}$ **cup shredded or finely chopped red cabbage**

$\frac{1}{2}$ **cup julienned or chopped yellow bell pepper**

$\frac{1}{2}$ **cup shredded carrots**

$\frac{1}{2}$ **cup alfalfa sprouts**

**1 cup mesclun greens**

Place the red cabbage, peppers, carrots, and sprouts in little piles forming a circle around the greens like a rainbow. Serve with Carrot-Ginger Dressing (page 114).

# Italian Salad (All Levels)

**MAKES 2 TO 4 SERVINGS**

**1 head romaine, chopped**

**2 cups arugula, chopped**

**2 yellow bell peppers, finely chopped**

**4 Roma tomatoes, chopped**

**4 sun-dried tomatoes, soaked and chopped**

**1 zucchini, julienned**

$\frac{1}{4}$ **cup fresh basil, chopped**

**2 tablespoons cold-pressed olive oil**

**1 tablespoon cloves garlic, minced**

**Celtic sea salt and freshly ground black pepper to taste**

Mix all vegetables in a large bowl. Dress with the basil, olive oil, sea salt, pepper, and garlic.

# Peace in the Middle East Salad
# (All Levels)

*If you love tabouli, you will love this dish!*

**MAKES 4 SERVINGS**

**1 cup halved cherry or grape tomatoes**

**½ cup English cucumber, chopped**

**¼ cup sweet onion, chopped**

**1 red bell pepper, chopped**

**½ cup fresh mint, chopped**

**½ cup fresh parsley, chopped**

**1 tablespoon cloves garlic, minced**

**1 tablespoon fresh ginger, minced**

**½ cup olive oil**

**2 tablespoons Nama Shoyu soy sauce**

**¼ cup lemon juice**

**1 tablespoon jalapeño, minced (optional)**

**¼ cup raw sesame seeds (optional)**

Mix all ingredients in a large bowl.

# Guacamole (All Levels)

*You may use this as a vegetable dip or spread it onto a vegetable sandwich.*

**MAKES ABOUT 2 CUPS**

**3 Hass avocados, chopped**
**Juice of 2 limes**
**1/4 cup finely chopped red onion**
**5 plum or vine-ripe tomatoes, chopped (or 1 cup grape tomatoes, sliced in half)**
**1/2 cup red or yellow peppers, diced**
**1/2 bunch fresh cilantro, chopped**
**Drizzle of olive oil**
**1 packet Splenda**
**Celtic sea salt to taste**

Mix all ingredients in a salad bowl.

# Guacamole Salad (All Levels)

*I cannot get enough of this salad. It's the kind of thing you can eat every night. Since avocados mix beautifully with sweet potatoes, you could round this salad off with a couple of them (topped with a touch of organic butter) for a fall or winter hearty, warm meal. Polish off the meal with a young coconut or some dark chocolate—or both!*

**MAKES 2 TO 4 SERVINGS**

**3 Hass avocados, finely chopped**
**4 ripe Holland tomatoes, diced, or 2 cups grape tomatoes, sliced in half**
**½ tablespoon garlic, minced**
**1 bunch cilantro, chopped**
**¼ to ½ pound baby romaine, mesclun, or regular romaine lettuce, chopped**
**Juice of 1 lime**
**2 tablespoons agave nectar (or 1 stevia packet)**
**Celtic sea salt and freshly ground black pepper to taste**

Mix all ingredients together and enjoy.

# Quick Guacamole Salad (All Levels)

**MAKES 1 TO 2 SERVINGS**

**3 heaping tablespoons Guacamole (page 127)**
**¼ pound baby romaine lettuce**

Place a couple of heaping spoons of guacamole atop a pile of baby romaine lettuce. It's simple and creamy-dreamy!

# Detox Salsa (All Levels)

*Try placing little mounds of this on your favorite raw crackers and breads to round out any raw salad or soup meal.*

**MAKES ABOUT 2 1/2 CUPS**

**8 Holland tomatoes, diced**
**1 bunch fresh cilantro, chopped**
**2 cloves garlic, chopped**
**1/4 cup sweet onion, chopped**
**Juice of 1 lime**
**1 jalapeño pepper, chopped**

Blend all ingredients in a large bowl and serve over salad or as a dip for raw veggies.

# Endive Bruschetta (All Levels)

**MAKES ABOUT 20 SERVINGS**

**3 Roma tomatoes, chopped**
**2 cloves garlic, chopped**
**1 cup packed fresh basil**
**2 heads endive, separated into leaves**
**Celtic sea salt and freshly ground pepper to taste**

In a mixing bowl combine the tomatoes, garlic, basil, salt, and pepper. Place a heaping tablespoon of the mixture on each endive leaf. This makes a sophisticated, fresh appetizer.

# Marinated Portobello Mushrooms
# (All Levels)

**MAKES ABOUT 2¹/₂ CUPS**

3 portobello mushrooms, stems removed and chopped into cubes

¹/₄ cup balsamic vinegar

3 tablespoons cold-pressed olive oil

3 tablespoons pure maple syrup

Celtic sea salt and freshly ground black pepper to taste

Mix all ingredients together and allow them to marinate for as few as 2 hours or as long as 2 days. This makes a great salad topper. I love to serve this dish over greens with the Raw Ceasar Dressing (page 112).

# Raw Goat Cheese Cabbage Sandwich
# (All Levels)

**MAKES 3 SERVINGS**

Dijon mustard

3 leaves red or green cabbage

6 thin slices Alta Dena raw cheddar-style goat cheese

Smear a small amount of Dijon mustard on each cabbage leaf and layer two slices of the goat cheese on top. Roll the cabbage leave into a tube and munch. It is the closest thing I have found to a raw cheese sandwich.

# Raw Caprese Salad

## (LEVELS 1D, 2D, 3, 4, AND 5)

*This salad offers all the pleasure of a real Caprese but without the gluey buffalo mozzarella clogging up your cells and pathways.*

**MAKES 2 SERVINGS**

**10 thin slices Alta Dena raw cheddar-style goat cheese**
**2 Holland or plum tomatoes, sliced about $\frac{1}{4}$ inch thick**
**10 leaves fresh basil**
**Drizzle of balsamic vinegar**
**Drizzle of olive oil**
**1 clove garlic, chopped**
**Celtic sea salt and freshly ground pepper to taste**
**1 teaspoon fresh ginger, diced (optional)**
**Sprinkle of stevia or Splenda**

Layer cheese slice, tomato slice, and basil leaf until each plate has five of each in the colors of the Italian flag. Whisk the balsamic vinegar, olive oil, garlic, salt, pepper, ginger, and stevia/Splenda. Spoon dressing on top of the salad.

# Beet "Prosciutto" (All Levels)

**MAKES 2 TO 4 SERVINGS**

1 large beet, thickly sliced on a mandolin
6 to 8 thin slices cantaloupe or 4 figs, quartered
Squeeze of lemon juice
Drizzle of olive oil
Celtic sea salt and freshly ground pepper to taste
Drizzle of agave nectar

Place the beet slices on a plate with the fruit on top. Add the lemon, oil, salt, pepper, and agave.

# Raw Neutral Pasta Pesto (All Levels)

*This is the only neutral pesto sauce I've ever seen, as it contains no nuts or cheese. You can put it on anything and mix it with anything—except fruit, but who in their right palate would do that?*

**MAKES ABOUT ½ CUP**

3 cups whole fresh basil
2 cloves garlic
5 teaspoons olive oil
1 teaspoon Celtic sea salt (or to taste)
1 large zucchini
2 Roma tomatoes, chopped

Blend basil, garlic, olive oil, and sea salt in a food processor. Turn zucchini into pasta with a Spiralizer, or finely julienne. Serve pesto sauce over the zucchini pasta. Garnish with chopped tomatoes.

# Simple Pasta Marinara (All Levels)

**MAKES 4 SERVINGS**

5 vine-ripe tomatoes

$\frac{1}{3}$ cup packed fresh basil

$\frac{1}{3}$ red bell pepper

$\frac{1}{4}$ cup fresh oregano (optional)

1 or 2 dates

1 tablespoon fresh ginger, minced

$1\frac{1}{2}$ cloves garlic

$\frac{1}{4}$ cup cold-pressed olive oil

2 shallots

$\frac{1}{4}$ cup red wine

$\frac{1}{2}$ cup sun-dried tomatoes

Celtic sea salt and freshly ground pepper to taste

1 large zucchini or spaghetti squash, cut into thirds

Place all the ingredients except zucchini in a blender and blend until creamy. Then, one at a time, place each of the zucchini pieces onto a Spiralizer and turn until all of the zucchini looks like angel hair pasta. If you do not have a Spiralizer, do not cut the zucchini into thirds, rather julienne it finely until it resembles long thin pasta strips. (Alternatively, you may use spaghetti squash.) Pour the tomato sauce over the zucchini.

# Kombu Pomodoro (All Levels)

*This is what I make when I'm craving the texture of real spaghetti.*

**MAKES 2 SERVINGS**

**12 ounces kombu seaweed noodles**
**2 Holland tomatoes, finely chopped**
**1 cup fresh basil, chopped**
**1 clove garlic, diced**
**1 tablespoon cold-pressed olive oil**
**1 tablespoon Celtic sea salt (or to taste)**
**Freshly ground black pepper to taste**

Rinse the kombu noodles in warm water to bring them to room temperature or above. Toss all the ingredients together and serve.

*Note:* Alternatively, you could make a cooked rendition of this—a very quick exit option—by using your favorite high-quality cooked marinara sauce (the Seeds of Change brand is excellent) in place of the raw tomato mixture, then top with steamed broccoli and even some raw goat cheese, if desired.

# Cooked Vegetables and Grain-Based Dishes

## Whole Wheat Lasagna

### (LEVELS 3D, 4, AND 5)

**MAKES 6 SERVINGS**

12 spelt or whole grain lasagna noodle strips, cooked al dente

25 ounces Seeds of Change pasta sauce

4 to 6 ounces Alta Dena raw goat cheese, grated or thinly sliced

1 clove garlic, chopped

1 zucchini, thinly sliced lengthwise on mandolin

1 eggplant, sliced lengthwise on mandolin

10 fresh spinach leaves

¾ cup packed fresh basil

Freshly ground black pepper to taste

Preheat the oven to 350°F. In a large baking dish, layer the lasagna strips, tomato sauce, most of the goat cheese, garlic, vegetables, basil, and pepper. Then add a final layer of the goat cheese. Bake for 25 minutes. This dish is excellent for easy entertaining. I serve it topped with a fresh basil leaf.

# Kamut Pasta Pomodoro

## (LEVELS 2D, 3D, 4, AND 5)

**MAKES 4 SERVINGS**

1 package kamut fusilli pasta, cooked al dente

6 large ripe tomatoes, diced

1 cup fresh basil, sliced into strips

1 clove garlic, minced

1 cup cold-pressed extra-virgin olive oil

Celtic sea salt and freshly ground black pepper to taste

Top the cooked pasta with with tomatoes, basil, garlic, olive oil, sea salt, and pepper.

# Simple Detox Pizza

## (LEVELS 2D, 3D, 4, AND 5)

*This is a favorite at my kids' play dates. Their friends love it!*

**MAKES 6 SERVINGS**

1 sprouted grain tortilla

3 tablespoons Seeds of Change pasta sauce

10 fresh basil leaves (optional)

2 ounces Alta Dena raw cheddar-style goat cheese, thinly sliced

Place the tortilla in a skillet. Spoon the pasta sauce evenly on the tortilla. Layer the basil on top of the sauce, and then sprinkle the cheese evenly on top of the basil leaves. Put pan over high heat and let the pizza cook until the cheese melts. Remove from the heat and slice like pizza.

# Detox Pizza #2

## (LEVELS 2D, 3D, 4, AND 5)

**MAKES 1 SERVING**

¼ cup Seeds of Change pasta sauce

1 sprouted grain pita or sprouted grain tortilla

1 cup any chopped vegetable

Basil leaves (optional)

Preheat the oven to 350°F. Place the sauce on top of the pita, then pile the vegetables on top and add basil if desired. Bake for about 15 minutes and serve hot!

# Detox Quesadilla

## (LEVELS 2D, 3D, 4, AND 5)

*This dish works great as an appetizer when you're entertaining the "uninitiated."*

**MAKES 6 SERVINGS**

3 sprouted grain tortillas

5 ounces Seeds of Change pasta sauce

4 ounces Alta Dena Raw cheddar-style goat cheese, thinly sliced

1 avocado, sliced

Place 1 tortilla in a skillet. Spoon the pasta sauce evenly over the tortilla and cover evenly with cheese. Top with a second tortilla. Layer the slices of avocado evenly, and finally top with the last tortilla. Cook over high heat until the cheese melts. Grill both sides until slightly brown. Remove from the heat and slice like a pizza. It's like a hearty "Big-Mac" quesadilla!

# Avocado-Vegetable Sandwich

### (LEVELS 2D, 3D, 4, AND 5)

**MAKES 1 SERVING**

**Romaine lettuce or baby greens**

**1 tomato**

**1 avocado, sliced**

**2 slices whole grain bread (such as Alvarado St. Bakery sprouted grain), toasted (optional)**

**Mustard, Liquid Gold Elixer (page 102), or Raw Caesar (page 112)**

**Vegetables (optional)**

Place the lettuce, tomato, and avocado between the bread slices. You may use mustard, Liquid Gold Elixir, or Raw Caesar to moisten. Add any other vegetables you like. Sprouts, cucumber, and sweet bell peppers are wonderful options!

# Portobello Sandwich

## (LEVELS 2D, 3D, 4, AND 5)

**MAKES 1 SERVING**

**1 portobello mushroom, sliced about ½ inch thick**

**1 cup vegetable broth**

**Dijon mustard**

**2 slices sprouted multi-grain bread**

**1 Holland tomato, sliced**

**¼ avocado, sliced**

**¼ cup baby lettuce**

Cook the sliced mushrooms in the vegetable broth until they are semisoft and cooked through. Place the desired amount of mustard on 1 slice of bread. Layer the tomato slices, mushrooms, avocado, and lettuce. Top with the mushrooms and the other slice of bread. Cut in half and enjoy!

# Sprouted-Grain Portobello Mushroom Fajitas

## (LEVELS 2D, 3D, 4, AND 5)

**MAKES 2 TO 4 SERVINGS**

**2 jumbo portobello mushrooms**

**3 tablespoons balsamic vinegar**

**4 teaspoons stone-pressed olive oil**

**2 Bermuda onions, thinly sliced**

**2 medium red bell peppers, thinly cross-cut**

**2 medium yellow bell peppers, thinly cross-cut**

**$1/4$ teaspoon chili powder**

**Celtic sea salt and freshly ground black pepper to taste**

**Four burrito-size sprouted grain tortillas (such as Alverado St. Bakery)**

**1 to 2 tablespoons Guacamole (page 127)**

**$1/4$ cup chopped tomatoes**

Rub the mushrooms with the vinegar and olive oil, then toss with the onions and peppers. Season with the chili powder, sea salt, and pepper.

Grill the mushrooms, onions, and peppers on a nonstick grill for 3 to 4 minutes on each side over medium heat. Remove from the heat. Warm the tortillas in the microwave. Slice the mushrooms in ½-inch bias cuts and arrange evenly on the tortillas with the peppers and onions on top. Fold the tortillas over the vegetable.

Serve the fajitas with guacamole and chopped tomatoes.

# Sautéed Vegetables

### (LEVELS 1D, 2D, 3, 4, AND 5)

**MAKES 2 TO 4 SERVINGS**

1 broccoli head, cut into mini florets

1 zucchini, sliced into coins

1 summer squash, sliced into coins

1 large carrot, julienned

½ sweet onion, diced

1 red bell pepper, julienned

2 cloves garlic, minced

6 to 12 ounces Pacific vegetable broth (as needed)

Place all the ingredients in a large skillet. Cook over medium heat until the vegetables reach the desired tenderness.

# Asian Brown Rice

## (LEVELS 2D, 3D, 4, AND 5)

**MAKES ABOUT 8 CUPS**

4 cups brown rice
1 tablespoon garlic, minced
1 tablespoon fresh ginger, minced
½ cup mirin
½ cup Nama Shoyu soy sauce

Bring the rice and 6 cups of water to a boil. Let it boil for 15 minutes, then simmer, uncovered, for another 15 minutes. Cover and remove the pot from the heat and let it sit for 10 minutes. In a small bowl, mix together the garlic, ginger, mirin, and Nama Shoyu, and pour over the rice. This is great with steamed or roasted vegetables and a great big raw salad!

# Pita Chips

## (LEVELS 2D, 3D, 4, AND 5)

**MAKES ABOUT 4 SERVINGS (40 CHIPS)**

2 whole wheat or sprouted grain pita bread
2 teaspoons organic butter
Sea salt and your favorite spices (optional)

Slice the pita in half so that you have two rounds. Preheat the oven to 350°F. Spread the butter over the pita, sprinkle with seasonings, if desired, and cut into about 10 mini triangle "chips." Bake pita chips until crisp, about 7 minutes. The chips taste great with vegetable soups!

*Note:* If you want sweet chips, use agave nectar instead of the spices.

# Cooked Flesh-Based Dishes

## Maple-Glazed Salmon

(LEVELS 1D, 2D, 3D, 4, AND 5)

*This is ideal for entertaining. It's so quick and easy to prepare while quite possibly the juiciest, most full-flavored dish your friends have ever enjoyed!*

**MAKES 4 SERVINGS**

1 cup Nama Shoyu soy sauce or tamari

1 clove garlic

1 tablespoon fresh ginger

$\frac{1}{2}$ teaspoon toasted sesame oil

1 cup pure maple syrup

4 fresh salmon fillets, well rinsed

Mix the soy sauce, garlic, ginger, sesame oil, and maple syrup in a blender. Spread the soy mixture over the fish evenly in a baking dish. Marinate the fish in the refrigerator for 1 to 24 hours.

Preheat the oven to 450°F. Bake the fish for about 18 minutes, or until fish flakes easily with a fork. Serve with the Sautéed Vegetables (page 141).

# Chilean Sea Bass with Creamy Port Sauce

### (LEVELS 2D, 3D, 4, AND 5)

**MAKES 4 SERVINGS**

**1 cup organic heavy cream**
**¼ cup port**
**4 fillets Chilean sea bass, black sea bass, or cod**

Preheat oven to 400°F. In a saucepan, mix the cream and port. Allow the mixture to simmer on medium-low heat for 10 minutes. Bake the fish for 28 minutes, or until fish flakes easily with a fork. Place the fish on a plate with your favorite vegetables and top with a generous portion of the sauce.

*Note:* For those of you who are still cooking meat for others, this sauce works beautifully on filet mignon as well.

# Shrimp Consommé

## (LEVELS 2D, 3D, 4, AND 5)

**MAKES 2 TO 3 SERVINGS**

10 fresh jumbo shrimp, peeled
1 onion, chopped
2 cloves garlic, chopped
1 carrot, diced
2 Roma tomatoes, diced
$\frac{1}{4}$ cup fresh parsley, chopped
$\frac{1}{4}$ cup sliced scallions
5 cups water
1 teaspoon cayenne pepper
Celtic sea salt and freshly ground black pepper to taste

Place all the ingredients in a soup pot. Bring to a boil and then reduce to simmer over low heat for 35 minutes. Enjoy with fresh greens and cilantro.

# Hungry-Girl Omelet

## (LEVELS 2D, 3D, 4, AND 5)

**MAKES 1 SERVING**

**4 free-range eggs**

**1 cup any vegetable**

**¼ cup onions, chopped**

**½ cup mushrooms, chopped**

**1 teaspoon butter**

**Several slices Alta Dena raw cheddar-style goat cheese, or your favorite soft goat cheese**

Whisk the eggs in a large bowl. Add the vegetables. Melt the butter in a skillet over medium heat. Add the vegetable mixture and cook until the egg becomes semifirm. Then layer the cheese slices onto the omelet. Fold and continue to cook until lightly browned on both sides and the egg is no longer runny. Enjoy with lots of fresh baby greens and Liquid Gold Elixir (page 102). Any low-starch vegetables will combine perfectly with this dish.

# Raw Desserts

## Simple Pecan "Pie" (All Levels)

**MAKES 1 SERVING**

**4 dates**

**4 pecans**

Open and pit the date. Place a pecan inside and enjoy!

# You-Must-be-Kidding Chocolate Sauce (All Levels)

**MAKES ABOUT 1¼ CUPS**

**1 cup pure maple syrup**
**6 tablespoons pure cocoa powder**

Blend the maple syrup and cocoa powder in a blender. Serve with long-stem strawberries for dipping, or pour over Raw Chocolate or Vanilla Ice Cream (pages 164 and 165) with walnuts and bananas for a classic banana split! It's recipes like this that make this lifestyle so rewarding!

# On the Road Again (All Levels)

*This is what I eat for dessert when I'm traveling. I can usually find bananas and lemon juice (in transit, as well as in restaurants), and I always bring dates and agave with me.*

**MAKES 1 TO 2 SERVINGS**

**Juice of ¼ lemon**
**Drizzle of either agave nectar or pure maple syrup**
**2 bananas, sliced**

Squeeze the lemon juice and nectar on top of the bananas. Follow this up with a few fresh dates, if desired.

# Dom Pedro (All Levels)

*This is slightly sinful since it calls for real whiskey, but it puts a raw smile on your face that's worth a thousand enzymes! A must for entertainers!*

**MAKES 1 SERVING**

**2 tablespoons whiskey**
**2 heaping scoops Raw Vanilla Ice Cream (page 165)**

Place the whiskey and ice cream in a wine goblet and stir.

# Lemon Ice (All Levels)

**MAKES ABOUT 2 CUPS**

**1 lemon (peeled)**
**1 cup ice**
**6 packets Splenda**
**Splash of fresh apple juice**

In the K-tec Champ HP blender (I highly recommend using this blender for all the ice creams, as you will need one that can crush ice effortlessly), combine the lemon, ice, Splenda, and apple juice. Blend on #4 of the K-Tec or on the highest speed of your blender until the desired creamy, thick consistency is reached. If the mixture is too runny, add more ice. If it's too icy to blend, add more apple juice or water. Serve immediately.

# Raw Chocolate Pudding (All Levels)

**MAKES ABOUT 2 CUPS**

**Meat of 2 coconuts (or ½ an avocado)**
**6 dates**
**4 tablespoons pure cocoa powder**

Blend all the ingredients in a food processor until smooth. Delicious!

# Cheesecake Pudding (All Levels)

**MAKES 2 CUPS**

**1 cup raw cashew butter**
**⅓ cup lemon juice**
**⅓ cup raw honey**
**4 dates**
**1 teaspoon vanilla extract**
**½ teaspoon Celtic sea salt**

Blend the ingredients until smooth and top with ground almond powder, if desired.

# Hot Chocolate (All Levels)

**MAKES 1 SERVING**

1 cup Pacific Almond Milk, or homemade nut milk

1 packet stevia or Splenda

1 tablespoon Green & Black pure cocoa powder

Mix all ingredients in a saucepan. Stir well and heat over medium heat until hot and cozy.

# Chai (All Levels)

**MAKES 1 SERVING**

1 cup almond milk

1 tablespoon pure maple syrup, or 1 packet Splenda or stevia

Sprinkles of nutmeg, cinnamon, and clove

Mix all ingredients in a saucepan and cook over a medium heat until hot. If you are using fresh, raw almond milk and wish to maintain the integrity of the enzymes, you may warm the mixture carefully over low heat, keeping it under 115°F.

# Coconut Water Cleanse (All Levels)

**MAKES 1 TO 2 CUPS**

**1 young coconut**

Using a cleaver, carefully open the coconut and stick a straw inside. Enjoy!

*Note:* see page 100 for tips on opening a young coconut.

# MASTERFUL CREATIONS

FOR *ALL* LEVELS WITH EMPHASIS ON LEVELS 1 AND 2;

ALL DISHES ARE 100-PERCENT RAW

## Fresh Herb Cucumber Rolls (All Levels)

**MAKES 2 TO 3 SERVINGS**

1 English cucumber, sliced into thin, wide strips on the mandolin

1 cup organic alfalfa sprouts or snow pea shoots

1 large carrot, julienned

1 red bell pepper, julienned

1 cup young coconut meat, julienned

½ avocado, sliced

1 cup fresh cilantro

Topping of olive oil, balsamic vinegar, or lemon juice

Celtic sea salt to taste

Place the cucumber slices horizontally in front of you so that they are all overlapping to make a gigantic roll. Then lay the vegetables and cilantro vertically onto the left side of the cucumber. Then roll the cucumber, starting from the left and enveloping the vegetables, moving all the way to the far right. Do this until you've used up all the ingredients. Then place the rolls on plates, drizzle olive oil, balsamic vinegar or lemon juice, and sea salt over the rolls. Serve as is, or dip in Raw Teriyaki Sauce (page 115).

# Simple Raw Sushi (All Levels)

**MAKES 8 ROLLS**

**4 sheets nori seaweed**

**4 romaine leaves**

**1 cup alfalfa sprouts**

**1 cucumber, julienned**

**1 carrot, shredded or julienned**

Place the nori sheet in front of you. Lay one leaf of romaine lettuce horizontally on top of the nori on the side closest to you. Lay the sprouts, cucumber pieces, and carrot pieces horizontally following the line of the romaine leaf. Carefully roll the nori around the vegetables, pulling it gently toward you as you roll it to make it nice and tight. Then, moisten the end of the nori farthest from you with some water and seal it like an envelope. Slice the roll with a sharp knife down the middle. Dip in the Raw Caesar Dressing (page 112), or any other detox dressing that you prefer.

*Note:* You can eat as much of this sushi as you like. It's light and refreshing! Add avocado to make it more filling.

# Arame Salad (All Levels)

**MAKES 2 SERVINGS**

2 ounces soaked arame seaweed

$\frac{1}{2}$ cup red bell pepper, chopped

$\frac{1}{2}$ cup pineapple, chopped

$\frac{1}{4}$ cup basil, sliced

$\frac{1}{4}$ cup Nama Shoyu soy sauce

3 tablespoons rice wine vinegar

2 teaspoons sesame oil (toasted, optional)

Mix all ingredients into a medium-size bowl and toss.

# Japanese "Rice" (All Levels)

**MAKES ABOUT 2 CUPS**

1 cup chopped parsnips

$\frac{1}{2}$ cup raw pine nuts

2 tablespoons raw honey

1 tablespoon rice vinegar

3 tablespoons Raw Teriyaki Sauce (page 115)

Pulse the parsnips, pine nuts, honey, and vinegar until the mixture starts to look like brown rice. Add the sauce and mix well. Serve alongside the Arame Salad (above) with some Simple Raw Sushi (page 153) for a Japanese entrée!

# Raw Old-Fashioned Homemade Soup (All levels)

**MAKES ABOUT 5 CUPS**

**1 avocado, chopped**

**3 ears sweet corn, kernels cut off cob**

**1 yellow or red bell pepper, chopped**

**½ cup soaked sun-dried tomatoes, chopped**

**1 cup soaked okra, chopped**

**10 Holland tomatoes**

**½ shallot**

**3 cloves garlic**

**1 tablespoon Nama Shoyu soy sauce**

**1 tablespoon curry powder (optional)**

**1 tablespoon Celtic sea salt**

**2 red bell peppers**

**4 dates**

**Freshly ground black pepper to taste**

In a large mixing bowl, place the avocado, corn, chopped pepper, sun-dried tomatoes, and okra. Set aside.

Blend the Holland tomatoes, shallot, garlic, soy sauce, curry powder (if using), salt, bell peppers, dates, and black pepper in a blender until smooth. Pour the blended mixture over the chopped mixture and enjoy.

# Thai Coconut Bliss (All Levels)

*This is my favorite raw soup recipe. I often serve it as a starter at dinner parties, where it is met with tremendous enthusiasm.*

**MAKES 2 TO 4 SERVINGS**

**1 cup sliced thinly shiitake mushrooms**
**3 tablespoons chopped fresh basil**
**½ cup fresh lime juice**
**1 teaspoon Celtic sea salt**
**Meat of 3 young coconuts**
**1½ cups coconut water**
**1 tablespoon fresh minced ginger**
**¼ cup olive oil**
**4 dates, pitted**
**1 tablespoon Nama Shoyu soy sauce**
**1 clove garlic**

Place the mushrooms, basil, ¼ cup of lime juice, and the sea salt in a small bowl. Mix well and set aside.

Blend the coconut meat, coconut water, ginger, olive oil, dates, soy sauce, the remaining ¼ cup of lime juice, and garlic in a blender until smooth. Pour the blended mixture into bowls. Garnish with the marinated mushroom and basil mixture.

# Thai Delight (All Levels)

**MAKES 2 TO 4 SERVINGS**

3 cups coconut water

$\frac{1}{2}$ tablespoon Nama Shoyu soy sauce or tamari

$\frac{1}{2}$ teaspoon Celtic sea salt

1 tablespoon sesame oil

$\frac{1}{2}$ tablespoon cloves garlic

1 tablespoon fresh ginger

1 tablespoon lemon grass (optional)

2 red bell peppers, thinly sliced on a mandoline

2 medium carrots, cut into matchstick slices

2 pieces baby bok choy, finely chopped

Meat of 1 or 2 coconuts, sliced into long, thin strips like noodles

In a blender, combine the coconut water, soy sauce, salt, sesame oil, garlic, ginger, and lemon grass. Blend on high until liquefied. Pour mixture over the raw vegetables and coconut strips.

# Cranberry-Beet Medley Salad (All Levels)

*The combination of fennel, parsnip, beet, and cranberry makes this dish taste sophisticated and comforting.*

**MAKES 2 TO 4 SERVINGS**

**1 bulb fennel, very thinly sliced on the mandolin and then julienned**
**1 cup parsnip, thinly sliced into coin shapes**
**1 beet, thinly sliced into coin shapes**
**¼ cup Liquid Gold Elixir (page 102)**
**¼ pound baby romaine lettuce**
**½ cup dried cranberries**
**Freshly ground black pepper to taste**

Place the fennel, parsnip, and beet in separate bowls and allow them to marinate in the Liquid Gold Elixir for about 1 hour. Place half the lettuce on each plate. Then place the marinated vegetables on top of the lettuce. Add a handful of cranberries and fresh pepper and enjoy!

# Raw Pad Thai (All Levels)

**MAKES 4 SERVINGS**

**3 cups shredded purple cabbage**

**2 large carrots, julienned**

**1 bunch cilantro, chopped finely**

**1 large zucchini, julienned**

**Meat of 3 young coconuts, sliced into long, thin strips like noodles**

**1 cup of Amazing Raw "Peanut" Sauce (page 116)**

**1/2 cup chopped raw cashews**

Mix the cabbage, carrots, cilantro, zucchini, and coconut strips in a large bowl and toss. Serve this mixture topped with 2 to 3 tablespoons of the sauce and a sprinkling of cashews.

# Rawviolis (All Levels)

**MAKES 2 SERVINGS**

¼ cup sun-dried tomatoes

1 parsnip

½ cup Raw Neutral Pesto (page 132)

15 leaves fresh basil

½ cup olive oil

1 teaspoon Celtic sea salt

1 clove garlic

4 dates, pitted

1 large beet, julienned

1 zucchini, julienned

Preheat the oven to 200°F. Soak the tomatoes in luke-warm water for about 10 minutes. Slice the parsnip on a mandolin very thinly crosswise to create thin disks (these are your rawvioli pastas).

Place some pesto inside two parsnip disks and repeat until you're out of parsnip and pesto. This should make about 15 rawviolis.

Make raw marinara sauce by blending soaked, drained tomatoes, basil, olive oil, salt, garlic, and dates until smooth.

Garnish each serving of 5 to 7 rawviolis with ¼ cup of julienned beets and zucchini. Place the rawviolis in oven with the door open about 4 inches for about 20 minutes, or until parsnips are warm and soft. Serve topped with the marinara sauce.

# Holiday G-Raw-Muesli (All Levels)

*This mixture will offer a taste of the holidays year-round.*

**MAKES 4 TO 5 CUPS**

**1 cup raw pecans or walnuts**
**1 cup chopped dried apples**
**1 cup raisins or dried cranberries**
**1 cup raw sunflower seeds**
**$\frac{1}{2}$ cup chopped raw almonds**
**Pinch of ground cloves, cinnamon, and nutmeg**

Toss the ingredients well and serve in place of nuts, or enjoy in a bowl with almond milk and maple syrup.

# Chocolate Shake (All Levels)

**MAKES 4 SERVINGS**

**$\frac{1}{4}$ cup pure cocoa powder (Green & Black brand is my favorite)**
**$\frac{1}{2}$ cup almond milk**
**1 young coconut (or $\frac{1}{8}$ avocado)**
**1 teaspoon vanilla extract**
**2 trays of ice**
**8 packets stevia or Splenda**

Blend all ingredients on high speed until creamy. Serve immediately.

*Note:* Warm a sliced banana in open oven with a drizzle of You-Must-be-Kidding Chocolate Sauce (page 147). Then, just before serving, place a dollop of the shake on top—yummy!

# Raw Cinnamon Apple-Pear Pie (All Levels)

*If you choose to make the crust, it will be soft. You may opt to serve this as an apple crumble instead of an apple pie.*

**MAKES 1 PIE**

1 Pecan-Date Pie Crust (optional; page 163)
3 Gala apples, very thinly sliced on the mandolin
2 Granny Smith apples, very thinly sliced on the mandolin
1 ripe pear, very thinly sliced on the mandolin
$\frac{1}{4}$ teaspoon ground cloves
$\frac{1}{4}$ teaspoon cinnamon
$\frac{1}{4}$ teaspoon nutmeg
2 packets Splenda
$\frac{1}{4}$ cup raisins
$\frac{1}{2}$ cup lemon juice
$\frac{1}{2}$ teaspoon vanilla extract

If desired, make pie crust to place fruit on. If not, place fruit directly on a pie plate.

Create one layer of apple, topped by one layer of pear, topped by another layer of apple. Then combine the spices, Splenda, raisins, lemon juice, and vanilla extract and pour over the pie. Refrigerate for at least 1 hour before serving.

# Pecan-Date Pie Crust (All Levels)

**MAKES 1 CRUST**

**6 dates, pitted**
**$\frac{1}{2}$ cup pecans, walnuts, or macadamia nuts**
**$\frac{1}{4}$ cup Pacific almond milk or fresh almond milk**
**$\frac{1}{2}$ teaspoon vanilla extract**
**$\frac{1}{4}$ teaspoon nutmeg**
**$\frac{1}{4}$ teaspoon cinnamon**
**$\frac{1}{4}$ teaspoon ground cloves**

Blend the dates, nuts, almond milk, extract, and spices in food processor until uniform (if it's still a little chunky in places, that's okay). Place the mixture in a pie pan; press firmly. Fill with raw pie filling of your choice.

# Raw Ice Creams

The following ice creams, if not consumed immediately, should be removed from the freezer for approximately 15 to 20 minutes before serving. They will harden in the freezer but will return to their creamy texture, if given time to become slightly soft again. I highly recommend using the K-Tec Champ HP high-powered blender to make these recipes.

Keep in mind that the raw ice creams combine well with raw vegetables, nuts, and dried fruit. Wait three to four hours after a properly combined flesh or starch meal before eating.

## Raw Chocolate Ice Cream (All Levels)

**MAKES ABOUT 4 CUPS**

3 bananas

3 tablespoons pure cocoa powder (I recommend Green & Black and Shiloh Farms)

2 tablespoons organic raw, unsalted tahini

8 packets Splenda or stevia

6 organic dates, pitted

3–4 cups ice cubes (about 14 cubes)

Place the bananas, cocoa powder, tahini, Splenda/stevia, dates, and ¼ of the ice in a K-Tec blender or other high-powered blender. Slowly add the remaining ice cubes as long as the mixture is flowing and blending well. You may have to run it two or three times to use up most of the ice. You need not use all the ice, just enough to make the mixture thick. You may also wish to use a little coconut water to facilitate blending.

# Raw Vanilla Ice Cream (All Levels)

*This is a divine rendition of regular vanilla ice cream.*

**MAKES ABOUT 4 CUPS**

**Meat of 3 young coconuts**
**1 tablespoon pure vanilla beans**
**1/2 cup pure maple syrup**
**4 cups ice cubes (about 14 cubes)**

Place the coconut meat, vanilla beans, maple syrup, and 1 cup of the ice in a K-Tec blender, or other high-powered blender. Add the remaining ice cubes as long as the mixture is flowing and blending well. You may have to run it two or three times to use up most of the ice. You need not use all the ice, just enough to make the mixture thick. You may also wish to use a little coconut water to facilitate blending.

# Raw Strawberry Ice Cream (All Levels)

*This is the most popular of all my ice creams. It's deeply satisfying.*

**MAKES ABOUT 4 CUPS**

**Meat of 2 young coconuts**
**2 bags frozen organic strawberries (Cascadian Farms)**
**8 packets Splenda or stevia**
**6 organic dates, pitted**
**1 teaspoon organic strawberry extract**
**4 cups ice cubes (about 14 cubes)**

Place the coconut meat, strawberries, Splenda/stevia, dates, strawberry extract, and 1 cup of the ice in a K-Tec blender, or other high-power blender. Begin blending on #4 or highest speed. Add the remaining ice as long as the mixture is flowing and blending well. You may have to run it two or three times to use up most of the ice. You need not use all the ice, just enough to make the mixture thick. You may also wish to use a little coconut water to facilitate blending.

# Raw Orange Sherbet (All Levels)

*This one is a personal favorite; it reminds me of eating rainbow sherbet as a kid.*

**MAKES ABOUT 4 SERVINGS**

**2 young coconuts**

**8 packets Splenda or stevia**

**6 organic dates, pitted**

**1 teaspoon organic orange extract**

**4 cups frozen, fresh-squeezed orange juice cubes (about 14 cubes)**

Place the coconuts, Splenda/stevia, dates, orange extract, and 1 cup of the juice cubes in a K-Tec blender, or other high-powered blender. Begin blending on #4 or highest speed. Add the remaining juice cubes as long as the mixture is flowing and blending well. You may have to run it two or three times to use up most of the juice cubes. You need not use all the cubes, just enough to make the mixture thick. You may also wish to use a little coconut water to facilitate blending.

# SAMPLE MENUS
# FOR ENTERTAINING

## Thai Menu

### Appetizer

Spring-in-Your-Step Rolls and Raw Teriyaki Sauce

### First Course

Thai Coconut Bliss

### Second Course

Raw Pad Thai

### Dessert

Vanilla Ice Cream served in coconuts or Dom Pedro
Green & Black or Dagoba dark chocolate and/or raw brownies

### Wine Recommendations:

This dinner is great with a full-bodied white wine. I love the California
Chardonnays by Toasted Head and Francis Ford Coppola.

# Italian Menu

## Appetizer

Endive Bruschetta

## First Course

Italian Salad or Gazpacho

## Second Course

Raw Pasta Marinara

## Dessert Course

Raw Ice Cream served with Blessing's Coconautti raw cookies
Green & Black or Dagoba dark chocolate and/or raw brownies

## Wine Recommendation:

Try a great, robust red wine. Francis Ford Coppola makes a stunning Merlot.

# Delicious Detox Sampler

## Appetizer

Sunshine Joy

## First Course

Ambrosia

## Second Course

Maple-Glazed Salmon with Sautéed Vegetables

## Dessert Course

Raw Chocolate Ice Cream topped with You-Must-be-Kidding Chocolate Sauce
Green & Black or Dagoba dark chocolate and/or raw brownies

### Wine/Beverage Recommendation:

Complement this meal with your favorite red or white wine such as the Francis
Ford Copola wines or fresh coconut water.

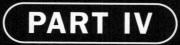

# PART IV

# REAL-LIFE SCENARIOS

# EATING OUT

You can eat out at any restaurant venue without getting derailed from your Raw Food Detox Diet lifestyle. While some restaurants will certainly be better options than others, if you are armed with a strategy, you can make consistent progress no matter where you are. In this section you will find solutions for restaurants ranging from fast-food chains to diners to five-star venues. While I certainly do not encourage frequenting low-end fast-food chains and dives, the reality is that this may still be an ingrained part of your lifestyle (perhaps because of your friends' or family's preferences). To cut you off completely from such eating establishments would be to exclude many of you from this dieting program—which is not at all the point!

No matter what your current lifestyle, you have every reason to find success on the Raw Food Detox Diet. My goal is to see as many of you succeed as possible—not just those with the lifestyle and financial means to get the highest-quality food easily. I firmly believe that, one day, this diet will be absolutely sustainable for all modern society. But to accomplish this, we need to step into the trenches of the fast-food chains and malls and offer up some new ideas!

Having said this, those of you who are still eating at fast-food restaurants should consider revisiting the reasons why you find yourselves at these places and start to cut back on your fast-food intake. Ultimately, your goal will be to avoid these venues entirely, but in times of early transition, they will not interfere with your cleansing as long as you stick to the following guidelines.

## TIPS FOR FAST-FOOD RESTAURANTS

While the Wendys' and McDonalds' of the world are not at the top of our desired venue list, you can always order a garden salad (lettuce, cucumbers, grape tomatoes, red onions, and carrots). If there is cheese sprinkled on the salad, remove it and do not use the dressing. I recommend carrying a container of your own dressing, such as the Liquid Gold Elixir (page 102). Alternatively, try to keep a lemon or stevia packets, and Celtic sea salt in your car or handbag for a quick-fix dressing as these don't need refrigeration. Avoid all fried foods, packaged dressings, and sodas. You may want to order two salads so you don't walk away hungry.

Keeping raw nuts, dried fruits, avocado, and bananas on hand would be a perfect way to round out a salad in this situation. You could top the salad(s) with any of these treats. If you choose the nut/dried fruits option, you could enjoy a raw treat or a Lara bar for dessert. If you choose the avocado, you could have a couple of bananas and/or some dates for dessert. You could even keep some herbal tea and natural sweetener among your stash, since you can always get hot water for a comforting herbal tea! You could also squeeze lemon into your water with stevia on a hot day for some quick lemonade.

# TIPS FOR OTHER CHAINS, STEAKHOUSES, AND UPSCALE RESTAURANTS

Chains like Applebee's and TGI Friday's offer better options. Believe it or not, even a Level 1 could eat comfortably at these places by topping a garden salad with a scoop or two of guacamole or a sprinkling of nuts and dried fruits. A Level 2 could order a garden salad as well as a plate of cooked seasonal vegetables or vegetarian fajitas (hold the tortilla, as it's probably made from white flour, and ask for extra guacamole instead). A Level 3, 4, or 5 could enjoy a great dinner of grilled salmon (hold the rice pilaf, garlic toast, etc.) with seasonal vegetables. You can always order extra sides of vegetables and entrée-size salads. Do note, however, that the various salads at these kinds of chains are not ideal in their original form. For example, a Tex Mex salad may include tortilla strips, guacamole, and cheese. You would have to order it with either the chicken or with the guacamole, but not both.

Now you might think that a steakhouse would be a huge challenge. Not so! I have found that steakhouses, with their no-nonsense approach to food, are actually among the easiest places to get good, cleanly prepared dishes. In addition to making heaping raw salads, they usually have good steamed vegetables—like broccoli, spinach, and carrots. I like to order a side of barbeque sauce for dipping!

Upscale restaurants are very easy, as you can always get a good mesclun salad (with goat cheese if desired) to start, and a great fish and vegetable entrée. For those of you who are vegan, vegetarian, or eating out at Level 1, you could order a steamed or light-oil sautéed vegetable entrée. When I do this, I order it with a large side of marinara sauce to pour over the vegetables to make it a really appealing, filling, and flavorful meal. In fact, when I go out to my favorite restaurant, I don't plan to eat an all-raw meal. On such nights, I eat somewhere between Level 1 and 3. Having this kind of leeway has been very effective at enabling me to stick with this diet for so long.

## ETHNIC RESTAURANTS: WHAT TO EAT AND WHAT TO AVOID

### What to eat at Chinese restaurants

- Steamed vegetables with steamed shrimp or chicken
- Steamed vegetables with brown rice (with a small amount of plum sauce, if desired)

### What to avoid at Chinese restaurants

- MSG
- Dumplings (white flour)
- Fried items
- White and fried rice
- Thick sauces
- Heavy meats (such as beef or pork, cheap cuts prepared in low-quality sauces)

### What to eat at Japanese restaurants

- Avocado, cucumber, or other vegetarian roll
- Sashimi (no rice)
- Fish entrée (no starch)
- Seaweed salad or house salad with ginger dressing
- Miso soup

- Japanese mixed vegetable plate

- Vegetable sukiyaki

## What to avoid at Japanese restaurants

- Fish rolls (combining flesh protein with rice)

- Soy products (occasionally they are okay but should not be consumed with regularity)

- Tempura

## What to eat at Italian restaurants

- Always begin with a mixed green salad with a natural vinaigrette

- Whole wheat pasta

- Marinara, puttanesca, tomato, or broth-based primavera sauces

- Grilled fish or other seafood

- Baked, grilled, or rotisserie chicken

- Vegetable plate (may contain some sautéed vegetables for extra flavor, but ask that only minimal amounts of oil are used)

## What to avoid at Italian restaurants

- Cream sauces

- White pasta

- White bread

- Gnocchi

- Breaded meats

- Starchy sauces

- Very oily vegetables

## What to eat at Indian, Thai, and Malaysian restaurants

- Curried vegetables or other low-oil vegetables

- Brown rice

- Any grilled, seared, or steamed seafood

## What to avoid at Indian, Thai, and Malaysian restaurants

- Fried or battered dishes

- White rice

- Poorly combined dishes

## What to eat at Middle Eastern restaurants

- Grilled vegetable kabob

- Baba ghanouj

- Whole wheat pita or vegetarian gyros

- Greek-style salad

- Tabouleh

- Hummus (for Levels 4 and 5)

- Grilled or seared fish or lamb

## What to avoid at Middle Eastern restaurants

- Meat gryros

- Yogurt

- Couscous

- Fried and battered dishes

# DINING AT PRIVATE HOMES, SOCIAL EVENTS, AND GATHERINGS

## BEING *GUEST*RONOMICALLY CORRECT

One of the most frequently asked questions I hear is, "What do I do when I'm a guest at someone's home?" This question is especially important during certain times of the year, when it may seem that you're spending more evenings at other people's homes than at your own.

I know it's not always easy to adhere to an eating plan when you're a guest at someone's home, but *you can always properly combine your meal*. There's almost always a vegetable dish and a salad. Typically, a flesh-vegetable focused meal will be the best choice, as starch options are rarely of the quick exit variety. Alternatively, you could bring a large, delicious salad, vegetable dish, or vegan soup to add to the menu. Just be sure to mention this (and the fact that you're on a diet) to the host or hostess ahead of time, and I'm sure he or she will be delighted. And don't forget to relish in the dishes that you can eat and tell the cook how wonderful they are!

While it's good to have a game plan for these occasions, the most important thing is to loosen up a bit on the reins. Make sure, first and foremost, that you are a good guest, and second, that you enjoy yourself. As any good host/hostess will tell you, part of being a good guest is enjoying yourself. Remember, you were invited because the host/hostess wants that special something that only you can bring to the gathering!

If you are planning to stay at someone else's home long-term, you should take the time to call and let them know they need not stock up on donuts and potato chips for you. If they insist on having something for you, let them know that you largely eat fresh fruits and vegetables and that you will be delighted to go to the store for them. Be clear about what you want. If you love oranges, say so. Friends and family want each other to be happy, so everyone will benefit if you speak up. You might also volunteer to go out to get breakfast for everyone in the morning, and in addition to picking up bagels and coffee for them, dash through the produce isle and get fruits, veggies, and anything else you might want for the day. Just be sure to get enough to share because your fresh produce will be irresistible to everyone! [At the end of your stay, it's always a good idea to offer a thank-you gift—perhaps a pint of homemade Raw Tahini Dressing (page 111) or Carrot-Ginger Dressing (page 114).]

Don't get hung up on dogma. The Raw Food Detox Diet is not about dogma. It is about making the best food choices you can under the circumstances. Let your instincts guide you to the healthier choices. If cooked vegetables and fish are all you can get, that's fine. You're still going to lose weight and move in the right direction. But by the same token, do not eat something you do not wish to eat out of some sense of obligation. If your friend is going to be mortally offended when you don't eat her crab cakes, that's her issue. Only eat outside the parameters of this diet if it's your choice to do so.

# CASUAL GATHERINGS LIKE BARBEQUES AND BUFFETS

These types of gatherings are generally easier than more formal meals. You usually have the option of bringing a dish and picking what goes on your plate, so load up on the good stuff and follow these tips:

- Always start the meal with a raw salad, which you can always bring with you even if you're the only one that ends up eating it.

- Enjoy plenty of *raw* corn. Cooked corn is a starch, but raw corn is neutral and may be enjoyed with both starch and flesh. It's sweet, crunchy, hydrating, and filling. If you like raw corn (as many people do), simply ask that a couple of cobs be put aside for you.

- Chicken, beef, and fish can all be safe options when cleanly prepared with, say, just a little barbeque sauce on the grill. Condiments like barbeque sauce, curry sauce, and even a little ketchup are not going to interfere with this diet unless you eat them on a daily basis.

■ Don't eat fruit after the meal. (If fruit is available early on, you may eat it as your first course.)

■ Bring a Green & Black 70-percent chocolate bar or a raw treat with you for dessert! (This also works great at weddings. I always take one with me to ensure I don't feel deprived.)

# PLANNING FOR THE HOLIDAY SEASON

## BE ARMED WITH A STRATEGY

We've all heard the statistic that the average American can easily pile on between 5 and 10 pounds over the holiday season. Many of you can vouch for that firsthand and are already dreading what another holiday will do to your waist-to-hip ratio. Without a concrete health strategy, you could easily have your diet "carpet-bombed" this holiday season. You can have all the best intentions, but if you're not braced with holiday meal solutions like the ones I am providing, you run the risk of backtracking with every holiday cocktail party, office party, and dinner party on your calendar. Know what you're going to eat, keep healthy snacks on hand, and plan ahead for guest appearances.

Based solely on habit, most of us stuff ourselves to the gills between Thanksgiving Day and New Year's Eve. In fact, we practically consider it our God-given right to overindulge during the holiday season, throwing dietary caution to the wind in favor of holiday cookies and eggnog. It all seems harmless enough, but such excess can create a domino effect on our health resulting in weight gain and a weakened immune system that can shut our body down for weeks with colds and flus.

There is no reason for you to feel deprived during the holidays on this program. You'll just need a different approach. Celebrate this holiday season with delicious, indulgent, but properly combined meals, balanced with fresh, raw fruits and vegetables. Here are practical, key tips that will enable you to avoid an agonizing post-holiday hangover at the end of it all. Believe it! Instead of waking up each day feeling sluggish and run-down by the gross amounts of heavy meals and sugary desserts you consumed in the previous weeks, you'll be able to rise and shine even leaner and healthier than you are today without missing a single party!

- **Strive for good food combinations**. Do not mix proteins and starches, and add lots of watery vegetables. This way you can eat to your heart's content without over-taxing your digestive system.

- **Choose the right starches.** Avoid refined starches such as white rice, white bread, potatoes, and white pasta. Permissible starches are sweet potatoes, whole grain bread, whole wheat pasta, brown rice, and other whole grains such as millet, wheat berries, and quinoa.

- **Keep raw treats handy throughout the season.** The best defense is a strong of-fense, so always be prepared with ultrahealthful raw snacks like bananas, dried un-sulfured fruit, raw nuts, and Goldie's Carob bars. This way, you won't automatically reach for the Christmas cookies or the chocolates your coworker brought to the of-fice just because you're "starved" or need a little pick-me-up.

- **Let your body recuperate after a heavy, ill-combined meal.** If you do wind up caving in and eating a heavy, ill-combined meal, the best antidote is to drink only freshly ex-tracted juices (such as a combination of carrot-romaine-celery-cucumber or any other veggie combination you like) and eat only fresh fruits throughout the following day un-til dinner. This will give your body a chance to digest and eliminate that large meal. (The worst thing you could do is eat *another* heavy meal that following morning or day.)

- **Enjoy your favorite fresh fruit for breakfast.** With so many heavy meals this season, the last thing you need is one more. Use the morning hours to give your body a break from digesting heavy foods, while supplying the enzymes, vitamins, and minerals it needs to function at peak level.

- **Eat lots of fresh greens with each holiday meal.** Green vegetables (especially leafy greens like mesclun, romaine, and spinach) are full of chlorophyll and live enzymes that will help break down those difficult-to-digest holiday foods—not to mention fill you up so you don't eat too much stuffing!

- **Take the time to enjoy your holiday meals and *never* eat under stress.** Holiday meals are not the time to bring up heavy family issues. Nothing could be worse for your digestion than feeling stressed. Make mealtime a joyous affair. Celebrating the company first and the food second (taking the time to chew your food well) will go a long way toward preventing overeating and indigestion.

- **Split your holiday feasts in two.** There is no reason you have to eat everything that's served on your plate in one sitting. To avoid overeating, try having the turkey and vegetable dishes one night, and the stuffing/starchy dishes with vegetables and greens the following night. Keeping your combinations simple will help prevent weight gain and sluggishness.

- **Have your pie and eat it, too.** If you keep your food combinations simple, avoid overeating, and make sure to eat some fresh greens with your meals, you can enjoy a little bit of your favorite dessert on a special occasion. If you're happy with your dark chocolate, that's even better!

- **Maintain control.** Don't make a bad meal worse. Often when we overeat we think, "Oh well, I've been this bad, I may as well have another piece of pie now." Before you know it, you've taken an only moderately damaging meal and created a major burden on the body. A little indulgence is okay. Don't let it cause you to careen out of control.

- **Drink minimally during mealtime.** When you drink large amounts of water with a meal, you dilute your precious digestive juices and your body needs to work that much harder to break the meal down. The more work a meal takes to break down, the less weight you will lose and the more sluggish you will feel.

# DIETING ON A LIMITED BUDGET

When you first start the Raw Food Detox Diet, it may seem costly, since you will need to restock your kitchen with some new items. However, once you've made the initial transition, maintaining your kitchen will be less expensive in the long run. When I was shopping at a traditional supermarket, I would spend an average of $800 per month on groceries. At that time, my husband and I were eating four to six meals out every week. I continue to spend an average of $800 per month on groceries, but now I prepare almost all of my family's meals, using the highest quality plant-based ingredients on the planet. What a difference!

Packaged food is very expensive, yet it appears that households with very low incomes tend to be the largest consumers of packaged products—and consequently the social sector suffering the most from obesity and diabetes. If you are on a budget, it simply makes much more sense to put your food dollars toward natural foods. You'll spend less on doctor visits, and you'll be naturally beautiful without having to spend a lot of money on makeup, clothes, facials, and other cosmetic purchases. In short, you don't have to be a millionaire to look like a million dollars!

This does raise an interesting comparison, though. For example, a container of raw almond butter costs about $8, whereas a container of store-bought peanut butter costs about $5. The almond butter is a far superior food because it provides essential raw enzymes, calcium, and protein that the body can fully assimilate, whereas the store-bought peanut butter is full of hydrogenated oils, salt, sugar, and other preservatives that the body cannot process. In the long run, isn't it worth spending those few extra dollars on the almond butter? It baffles me that people think $3 is too much to spend on a papaya, but they'll spend that amount or more on a bag of potato chips and a soft drink! Raw granola costs $8 a bag, whereas the cooked variety costs about

$5.50. For an extra $2.50 you are getting a food that can actually exit the body—not weigh it down.

For those of you on a very tight budget, it will be easy for you to eat economically at Levels 3 to 5. Whole grains like millet, brown rice, and wheat berries cost very little and are very filling, as are sweet potatoes and sprouted grain breads. You can buy fresh fruits and vegetables as well as many raw nuts and grain items at inexpensive co-ops. And the Kollar cookies are also very reasonably priced.

At Levels 1 and 2, where the desire for gourmet raw food and specialty raw food treats (like raw pecan pie bars, raw breads, and raw brownies) kicks in, your budget will go up. But if you like simple foods and are creative with nuts, dried fruit, and dates, you can keep costs down.

Just do your homework, price things out online, and you will find a way to fit this dieting lifestyle into the tightest budget. Another approach is to see where you're spending money needlessly. Manicures and pedicures are not necessities. Impulsive long-distance phone calls and expensive coffees should take a backseat to the pure bliss of cultivating a clean body! Cut back on other expenses if you must, and learn to put your health and well-being first.

## Inexpensive Transition Foods

> Carrot soup and other vegetable soups
> Sweet potatoes
> Sprouted grain bread products
> Brown rice and other whole grains
> Kollar cookies (www.kollarcookies.com)

## Inexpensive Raw Food Products

> Raw almonds and walnuts
> Organic raisins and apples
> Banana and almond butter shakes
> Tahini-based salad dressings and shakes
> Avocados
> Dates
> Dee Dee's raw snack items (see appendix)

# THE OFFICE

I have worked with enough business people and office personnel to know that this program can be successful in any office setting. Here are a few key tips for adapting the program to your office lifestyle:

- Bring a bag of fresh fruits into the office every day. I recommend bananas, grapes, figs, and other no-mess fruits. One of my favorite fruit tricks is to bring a whole cantaloupe to the office. Keep a sharp knife and a metal spoon in the kitchen or in your desk drawer. Cut the cantaloupe in half, remove the seeds, and—voila—you have two bowls of fruit. Breakfast is solved.

- Double the recipe of your favorite raw dressing. Put half in your refrigerator at home and the other half in your fridge at the office. This way you can always enjoy a large satisfying salad for lunch.

- Keep nuts, dried fruit, and raw treats in a file drawer. They do not need to be refrigerated if eaten within two weeks. Also keep handy your favorite sweetener, Celtic sea salt and/or Spike brand seasoning.

- Have a plan for office gatherings, like when everyone is eating cake to celebrate a birthday, an engagement, or an office baby shower. Have a supply of herbal tea, Splenda, and a favorite mug, so that you'll have something to take with you to these gatherings. Any 70-percent chocolate is also great to have on hand for such occasions.

■ Take responsibility for your body and learn to say "no." Just because you used to go with your colleague for a frozen yogurt every day at three o'clock or for a drink and a snack after work, doesn't mean you can't change those habits. Sure, your colleague might find it disconcerting at first, but he/she will get over it. Don't take a cookie just because it's there or someone says you should. Likewise, don't beat yourself up if you do take one. Just be very cognizant of when you are acting out of old habit rather than transitioning responsibly.

# TRAVELING

One of the most challenging times to stick to a healthful eating program is when you're traveling. Since many of you travel, it's often critical to have a set of travel rules and tools in place. The holidays are a particularly busy travel season. But whether you are traveling by ship, plane, or train, the strategy is the same: *plan ahead!*

## BASIC TRAVEL TOOLS

If you are flying before three o'clock in the afternoon, eat nothing but fresh fruit and fresh juices before your flight. This will keep your system clean and hydrated so that you won't be affected as much by dehydration and constipation when you arrive at your destination. Then pack 2 bananas (or other fruit), 1 to 2 avocado sandwiches, and a whole grain cookie. Enjoy the bananas if you're hungry early in the flight. The avocado sandwiches will come in handy when the meals are passed out. You will have something truly delicious to enjoy and a yummy cookie to top it off. For those of you who eat "raw till dinner," bring additional fruits, dried fruits, and/or a chopped salad with you on the flight. Avoid airplane food at all cost—yes, even if you're traveling first class! The only exceptions to this rule are plain green salads and the possible addition of first-class grilled chicken *or* a first-class whole grain roll.

If you are flying after three o'clock in the afternoon, eat fruits until lunchtime. At which time you may either have an all-raw meal such as a large raw salad with avocado, a grain-based meal like a vegetable sandwich, or lentil soup with a large salad. If you're stuck in the airport, you can always find a large salad and a couple of bananas. It is important to eat heartily at this point since it will be at least three hours until your next meal. Take bananas, apples, a vegetable sandwich, and a whole grain cookie to enjoy throughout the flight, if it is a long one. Remember to wait three hours after a meal before eating fruit again and thirty minutes after eating fruit before eating concentrated foods like grains, nuts, or flesh. Invest in some good plastic containers (and plastic utensils) for carrying chopped fruits, salads, sandwiches, and other lifesaving goodies.

Whether you are going away for four days or four weeks, take a quick trip to your local health food store for your favorite dried fruits, raw nuts, and raw snacks. I never travel without a stash of dried apples and my favorite raw treats—like the Lara bars, which my husband and kids wind up eating. (Lara bars are prepackaged, require no refrigeration, and are perfect when you want a filling snack.) Macadamia nuts and raisins are great to have on hand to add to your large raw salad at a poolside lunch or when you need a little energy boost for that last ski run. *Note:* when you are taking nuts or raw food treats to a warm climate, refrigerate these items as soon as possible to prevent them from going rancid.

## ADDITIONAL TRAVEL TIPS

- While you may not be able to get your green juice when traveling, you'll always be able to start your day with a fresh fruit plate and, in most cases, a freshly squeezed citrus juice. I typically ask the waitress (or room service) to bring me a couple of bananas, which I can snack on if I get hungry throughout the morning.

- Just before you check out of your hotel, order 1 to 2 vegetable sandwiches on whole grain bread from room service. Ask them to pack the sandwiches well, as you'll be taking them on the plane with you. Have them double-bag the paper bag that they use, just in case!

- When traveling, you are thrown out of your routine. This is what makes traveling so invigorating and mind-opening. However, it can also throw your body out of whack if you don't apply a good game plan, like the tools and tips listed above. Having said this, don't be so strict that you miss out on opportunities to try new things. Clearly, it takes a little extra effort to travel prepared but feeling great and having a delicious, healthful airplane snack makes it worth the effort.

## HOTELS AND SMALL TOWN RESTAURANTS

I've traveled all over the country and have never stayed in a hotel where I haven't been able to get a large, fresh fruit plate, a couple of bananas, and freshly squeezed grapefruit or orange juice in the morning. On the day that you're traveling, ask room service to include a well-packed whole grain vegetable sandwich with a side of mustard or a large raw salad for lunch, which they can bring at the same time that they deliver your fruit plate.

It is always easy to get a raw vegetable salad, whole grain toast with avocado, or grilled fish with steamed vegetables in a hotel—or at any restaurant in the area for that matter. Just be mindful of proper food combinations, and you can't go wrong.

I have traveled extensively eating this way and have found that I don't get sick when I travel on airplanes like I used to. (I used to think it was inevitable that I would catch a cold or something worse every time I traveled.) Eating this way also helps you to avoid dehydration, constipation, and headaches. And you'll suffer less from jet lag and general fatigue.

Last but not least, I highly recommend taking a Cara enema kit with you when you travel. If your eliminations slow down at all, it will come in handy!

# DETOX YOUR KITCHEN

You should detoxify your kitchen as soon as possible upon embarking on the Raw Food Detox Diet. The following is a "how to" list for preparing your kitchen for this lifestyle:

- Remove all the food from your kitchen and place it on the dining room table.

- Thoroughly clean (or hire someone to clean) your kitchen, including all the cupboards and the inside of the fridge.

- Discard or give to your local Foodbank all packaged goods that are not specific to the program. This includes all canned products, packets of sugar-free hot cocoa, bullion cubes, crackers, chips, and all the other scary stuff that may have been lurking in your kitchen. If you have family or a roommate who will not be dieting, or if you want to save certain items for guests, you may create shelves in your cupboard and fridge for that purpose. Sectioning shelves in this way will remind you that such items are off limits for your own goals and purposes.

- Segregate your cupboard and fridge into four categories: (1) approved starches, sprouted grains (all sprouted grain products must be kept refrigerated; they also store beautifully in the freezer), kamut or other whole grain pasta, Kollar cookies, legumes, grain crackers, and so forth. (2) flesh and dairy products like raw goat cheese, butter, cream, fish, and so forth. (3) raw nut and dried fruit products like raw treats, raw nuts, seeds, dried fruits, and so forth. (4) neutral products like condiments, broths, seasonings, and so forth.

- Every time you go shopping—until making smart food combinations becomes a no-brainer—place your new purchases in their rightful categorical spot.

# DETOX YOUR BATHROOM

You might not think your toiletries are sabotaging your health and beauty, but consider this: everything you put on your skin is absorbed into your bloodstream. That includes soap, shaving cream, body lotion, deodorant, mouthwash, toothpaste, makeup, and any other products you may be using. No, I'm not suggesting that you grow your leg hair, stop using deodorant, or go to work without wearing any makeup. However, it's high time we took a look at the hazardous ingredients in mainstream bathroom products. Just as it's your decision to make certain dietary changes, it's up to you to decide whether to switch one or two natural alternatives or to throw out all your drugstore products at once and adopt a whole new, natural arsenal. Any small change in this department will be significantly beneficial.

## STEPS FOR DETOXIFYING YOUR BATHROOM

- Remove all your bathroom products—from the medicine cabinet to the bathtub to that scary place under the sink!

- Thoroughly clean (or hire someone to clean) the bathroom.

- Throw away any products that you simply don't use, including old bottles of prescription medication, old mini hotel shampoos, old make-up that's been outdated in more ways than one, and anything that you have trouble identifying.

- Arrange like products together (i.e., hair products with hair products, makeup with makeup).

- Now look at the ingredients in your products. Does your soap contain lye? Does your toothpaste or mouthwash contain ethanol sodium fluoride, sodium saccharin, or yellow dye #5? If you use an antiperspirant or deodorant, does it contain ammonia, formaldehyde, phenol (known carcinogens), or triclocarban (a suspected cancer-causing agent with daily use)? Does your shampoo or conditioner contain cocamide DEA or methylisothiaolinone (other carcinogens and mutagens)? Does your shaving cream contain a-pinene? Other suspects to look out for include talc, mineral oil, aluminum, polyvinylpyrrolidine (typically found in hairspray), phenol carbolic acid, PEG-40, padimate O, and the preservative BNPD (typically found in sunscreen).

- Determine which of these products you think you could live without and then select natural alternatives to them from brands like Avalon Organics, Jason's, Young Living, and many others that are available at natural markets like Whole Foods.

- Clean the items you decide to keep before restoring them to their rightful place.

- Gradually replace carcinogenic toiletries with the natural ones that you like. You may be surprised by how much you prefer the natural products. (I don't miss the drugstore items at all.)

Also keep in mind that, as you begin to apply your new dietary principles, you simply won't need to use so many beauty products. You will naturally begin to have better breath (eliminating the need for mouthwash), your skin will become more even-toned and radiant, and your body odor will become less offensive.

You may decide that there are one or two things that you want to keep. In my case, I decided to be relaxed about makeup. First of all, I don't need to wear it every day. Second, I've removed so many hazards from my diet and the bathroom that my body can deal with just one or two synthetic beauty products (remember the "triage" system). So while I held onto my makeup, I got rid of every other offender. You see, the point is not to become a hippie and stop shaving your legs and armpits or dress exclusively in organic cotton and Birkenstocks. The point is to lift the burden of hazardous materials off your body so that it can fight all the other daily pollutants that you cannot (in most cases) control or even see.

It is also a good idea to find a high-quality face and body care line. Many face and body care lines claim to be natural, but one peek at the ingredients often shows that they're not. Beyond the age of twenty, everyone should take extra special care of their facial skin. A quality cleanser, exfoliant, toner, eye cream, and (most importantly) hydrating moisturizer should be your staples. After many years of sampling products, there are two cosmetic lines that I recommend the most: Renewal Vine Therapy (www.vinetherapy.co.za) and ERBE (212-966-1445; www.*erbedermocosmetica.com*). They offer the best antiaging cream!

# DETOX YOUR WARDROBE AND LIVING SPACE

Detoxifying your body leads to an overwhelming desire to clean and clear your living space. Getting rid of the clutter in your body will make you more aware of how much clutter is around you—in your household, at your office, or in your study space. Go with this natural inclination and start detoxifying your living space as soon possible. It will actually help your dieting efforts. When your living space is chaotic, you're less inclined to eat carefully. In fact, the clutter may actually drive you back to your bad habits, since people tend to eat when they want to avoid a task. On the other hand, an organized, beautiful living space will inspire you to keep a clean, beautiful body as well.

When changing your dietary habits, it is helpful to consider every aspect of your life that isn't quite working. For many of you, your living space ranks near the top of that list. All the clutter in your living and working space translates into clutter in your mind, heart, and emotional space. By clearing out the junk and making your space a highly functional part of your life, you and your body will be all the more inclined to follow suit.

I had the good fortune of meeting the highly regarded wardrobe stylist and closet expert, Eleanor Estes, at a time when I knew my home required serious reorganizing. Like most people, I wasn't particularly messy, but I fell into lazy patterns that created disorder in almost every area of my home. The first thing that she and I tackled was my wardrobe—her specialty!

The very first thing she had me do was take every item of clothing out of my closet. Then, one by one, I put each piece of clothing on. Based on simple criteria (Is this high-quality fabric? Does it fit properly? Is it dated?), we created two piles of clothing: one that would be given away, and one that would be properly organized and looked after.

To my surprise, we mutually agreed that more than 75 percent of the clothing I was holding onto would better serve a charity. First of all, most of my pants fell from the waist—a cut that typically hugs the hips in unflattering and dated ways. I quickly learned from Eleanor that pants should fall from the hips so that the pants drop in a clean line along the leg. She also pointed out that most women buy their pants a size too small. It's true, we always want to buy the smallest size that we can squeeze into, when the next size up is much more slimming!

In the end, I was left with the best clothing in my closet—the only clothing in my closet that I should have been wearing, according to Eleanor. Why would I ever want to be seen in less than flattering gear, anyway? The extra mounds of poorly fitting, dated clothing I was holding onto "just in case I needed them" went to people who really needed them, via various local churches. I never even missed those clothes.

Do you ever feel like you have a closet full of clothes but nothing to wear? Millions of people experience this every day. Yet, according to Eleanor, most people wear 20 percent of their wardrobe 80 percent of the time! By giving away the clothes that do not work in your life, you can then see what does work and what you need to make your wardrobe work for every occasion. Put your own clothes to the test. If an item of clothing matches any of the following criteria, it is time for you to get rid of it:

- You haven't worn it in over a season. (You can make exceptions for classic evening wear, high-quality classics, and sentimental favorites—to be placed in a sentimental box).

- It is permanently stained.

- It is torn beyond repair.

- It makes you feel bad about your body.

- You're saving it for when you lose 10 pounds. (You'll want to buy something new once you lose the weight. But if you really want to save this item, add it to your sentimental box and revisit it in three months.)

- You bought it only because it was on sale. (Remember, all you bargain hounds: a bargain is only a bargain when it is in style, fits, and works with what you already own.)

Once I picked out the clothes I wanted to keep, I divided them into two categories: fall/winter and spring/summer. Since it was spring, I put the fall/winter garments into newly purchased storage boxes and stored them under my bed. The spring/summer garments were placed on new *wooden hangers* (a must, according to Eleanor, because they do not compromise the shape of the clothing). I had creased so many clothes using plastic and wire hangers that I couldn't wear them until they were cleaned or ironed again—which was a terrible waste, but not something I would ever again have to tolerate.

## WARDROBE POINTERS FROM ELEANOR ESTES

- Store dressy shoes, evening bags, fancy hose, and special jewelry together in a clear shoebox, so they are protected and easy to locate when you need them.

- Categorize your drawers. Put undergarments, socks, pantyhose, pants, T-shirts, turtlenecks, costume jewelry, and workout clothes in separate drawers. Weed out items as you sort and organize.

- Save time by separating hosiery by color and storing each color in its own clear, plastic bag.

- Wherever possible, install hooks on the inside of closet doors.

- Store your clothes according to season—you can keep your "off-season" items in large, airtight plastic boxes under your bed.

- Organize your clothing according to type (shirts, pants, skirts) and color (dark to light)

- Keep several baskets in your closet for laundry, dry-cleaning, and mending. Don't hang anything that you can't currently wear.

- Store your shoes on a rack—either on the floor of the closet or on the back of the door—to keep them paired together and in good condition.

- If you have a lot of folding clothes, install some open shelves, bins, or a drawer system in your closet for easy access.

If you make sure that you return items where they belong in the closet, you will always keep it organized. If you never use your closet or keep it empty, you will not be making the best use of your space. If you perform daily minimum maintenance in your closets, you'll save yourself a lot of time and clutter in the long run—which is integral to the Raw Food Detox Diet lifestyle!

# RAISING A FAMILY: THE ULTIMATE REAL-LIFE SCENARIO!

The beauty of the Raw Food Detox Diet is that you can really keep it simple if you so choose. It doesn't require any more time than usual in the kitchen. The best way to manage family meals, if you are the only one eating this way, is always to make something that you can eat as part of the dinner. For example, if your family likes a flesh dish as part of their meal, broil, bake, or roast that item so you can also enjoy it with a large raw salad. If you would like to skip the flesh dish (depending on your detox transition level), simply prepare sweet potatoes or another high-quality starch dish that you can eat with your salad and that your family can enjoy with other foods (you might do this most of the time). It only takes a moment to pop a sweet potato into the oven. Once your family tries the Seeds of Change brand of seven grain pilaf, I doubt they'll ever ask for Rice-A-Roni again!

## HELPING YOUR TEENS AND TOTS

If you're a parent who wants your children to eat more healthful foods or lose weight, you can safely incorporate many elements of this diet in their lives. In fact, your children will fare better on this diet than on a low-calorie or low-fat diet because they will eat to satisfaction and not equate dieting with torture. Calorie-restrictive diets are not only hard for children to stick to but can be detrimental to their proper growth. The only one way to help children and adolescents stay slim without threatening their proper development is to change the way parents and children think about food. Your support is critical; you cannot expect your children to change their eating habits without also submitting yourself to a healthful program. As a parent, you must set the example!

Much like the average adult, the average teenager who is coming from a soda and fast-food lifestyle must be approached in a carefully gradational way. This is important for two main reasons. First, most adolescents laugh at the concept of "health food" and are automatically inclined to despise the food as a threat to their freedom. Second, if they transition too quickly, they will experience symptoms associated with cleansing (such as headaches, pimples, and indigestion). A young person won't want to put up with those symptoms, especially if they come on severely. There is also a third reason: many adolescents who have seen their parents yo-yo diet will just dismiss it as another fad and won't give it the respect it deserves.

The goal here is *not* to make a young raw foodist of your child. Nor is it important that he or she combine foods perfectly. The goal is simply to start upgrading the quality of the food that you keep at home—and, ideally, for school lunches. If you have a youngster just starting out, here's what you can do to start the transition:

- Get him/her to drink at least one glass of freshly squeezed orange or grapefruit juice first thing in the morning—on an empty stomach.

- Make a smoothie of banana, dates, organic frozen strawberries, orange juice, and a little romaine lettuce (they won't taste it) for him/her to enjoy in the morning or between school and dinnertime.

- Keep fresh-cut fruit in the fridge—kids will eat it!

- Exchange mainstream chips for the Guiltless Gourmet variety or the Olive Oil brand sweet potato chips.

- Start using whole grain bread (or sprouted grain, if your child will eat it).

- Replace peanut butter with raw almond butter. (There is no sweetness to raw almond butter, so you'll want to mix it with raw honey in many instances.)

- If your child has had calorie restrictions in the past, discourage it now. Explain that if he/she chooses these higher quality foods, there will be no need for calorie counting.

- Make your teen a glass of carrot-apple juice once a day for enzymes.

- Make a fabulously rich dip like the Guacamole, Raw Tahini Dressing, or Amazing Raw "Peanut" Sauce for dipping carrots and sweet peppers before dinner (see recipe section).

- Make cheese melts with the Alta Dena cheddar-style raw goat cheese and sprouted grain bread for snacks.

- Make Hot Chocolate (page 150).

- Get an air popper for popcorn and melt organic butter and sea salt on top.

- Make mealtime "family time." No television program or homework assignment is more important than learning how to relate to each other. Kids need this down time. Don't discuss anything stressful; just enjoy one another's company. This way, you will be nourishing your whole family both physically and emotionally.

- Make dinnertime fun by lighting candles and playing some relaxing music. You need to show that nothing is more important than family time to ensure that your child's priorities are well placed.

- Replace mainstream candy bars with organic pure chocolate bars, like the ones made by Dagoba and Green & Black.

After a while, or if you have already raised your child on a healthful diet, you can step up your efforts with the tips that follow:

- Eliminate all white pasta, bread, and other white grain products.

- Eliminate all packaged goods and substitute them with the transition foods.

- Use only raw nut butters in place of peanut butter.

- Use only whole wheat or kamut/spelt pastas.

- Prepare most of your family's dinners yourself.

- Encourage your child to make vegetable-fruit juices with you.

- Give your child fresh fruit or a fresh fruit smoothie first thing in the morning.

- Only use whole grain cereals (try Health Valley, Barbara's, or Cascadian Farms)

- Allow your child the occasional treat, like a real ice cream cone, but not the packaged frozen desserts that are chock-full of food coloring and hydrogenated fats.

- Let your child get excited about food preparation by having him or her take part in shopping and cooking.

- Let your child choose from an assortment of healthful transition foods for lunches and snacks.

- Keep grapes, organic apples, and cut fruit within easy reach.

- Put out a platter of your kid's favorite vegetables for dipping in his/her favorite raw dressing before dinner. Better yet, take it to your kid when he/she is doing homework or spending time with friends. (I've discovered that girl study groups love this!)

- Make plenty of spelt cookies.

If your child is happy living this way, you can also try these ideas:

- Introduce your child to Green Lemonade (page 101) as early as possible (from six months of age on). Both of my kids gladly suck it down by the glassful.

- Feed your child almost exclusively natural, detoxifying foods.

- Allow your child to enjoy sweet potatoes, sprouted grain bread products, whole grains, goat cheese, organic eggs, organic fish, and even the occasional grass-fed lamb chop. There's no need to encourage an all-raw diet; your child should generally be eating at a Level 2 or 3.

- Include two or three different types of fresh fruit in school lunches, in addition to a fruit smoothie or fresh juice in the morning.

- Let your child try raw granola with almond milk and raw honey (or maple syrup) as an anytime snack or meal. (My daughter loves to find this in her school lunch bag!)

- Keep lots of raw treats on hand for snacks. (My daughter loves the Raw Bakery 99.9-percent brownies and Lara bars.)

- Let your child help you make salads, soups, and raw dishes. (Both my kids love to stand up on chairs next to me when I chop the salad and taste every vegetable I cut up.)

- If your child is eating at this level, mealtimes need to be more flexible because he/she will be eating from natural hunger, not from stimulation or addiction. Encourage your child's "grazing," as it is the ideal way for growing children to eat.

Kids that comply with eating in this way should not be restricted from eating specific foods at special occasions—like birthday parties, holidays, or weddings. They must be permitted to have a slice of pizza or a piece of real birthday cake now and then. The irony is that, while they will be titillated by the idea of this foreign food, they probably won't be inclined to eat much of it. In the grand scheme of family life, these exceptions mean nothing. I always allow my kids to participate in the "food fun." Holding them back would only result in negative food associations and rebellion down the road.

## Set a healthy example for your child, and save him/her from the perils of an eating disorder

Many of you are mothers of teens and preteens who are already preoccupied with their weight. Understandably, you might worry that being too focused on your diet will send the wrong message to them. But there's no need to worry; in fact, learning how to eat healthfully is a great way for children and teens to avoid eating disorders. One of the main reasons that people develop eating disorders is to gain control. The typical thought process goes something like this: *If I can control my body, then I will be able to have control over something in my life.* The trouble with this perspective in an adolescent or preadolescent (more common in girls) is that the body is changing so quickly that it's natural, at that age, to feel out of control. It doesn't help that the media is filling young brains with images of skinny models and performers.

By adopting the program for yourself and your family, you will be showing your child that she can have more control over the health and beauty of her developing body by eating whole, natural foods than by any type of restrictive eating, bingeing, or purging that she might be considering. It is never too soon to educate our daughters (and our sons) about the importance of eating a diet that's high in natural plant foods. By doing this and emphasizing the cleanliness of the body, you may well be saving your child from a lifelong battle with weight, self-image, and health.

I do want to emphasize that you should *not* tell your child that you are on this detox program to lose weight. Instead, explain that processed, unnatural foods are not making you feel good and that you have learned a new way of eating that will make you feel much better and healthier. The weight loss and aesthetic results will soon be obvious and will appeal to him/her. Never pressure your child to eat as you are; let the natural foods speak for themselves, and only tell him/her more if he/she asks you about it directly.

The most effective way for a parent to prevent a child from developing an eating disorder is to expose him/her to a large variety of fresh fruits, vegetables, nuts, nut butters, and food preparations from a very young age. By doing this, your child will develop a natural taste for these healthful foods and will avoid the emotional and physical consequences of being overweight. I firmly believe that a child who eats according to this program will never develop a weight problem.

## TEENS AND TOTS MENU IDEAS

Your teens and tots can enjoy just about any food using natural ingredients. For example, if they want popcorn, make them some air-popped popcorn with melted butter and sea salt. Try making pancakes and French toast from scratch, using organic eggs, spelt flour (for pancakes), and sprouted grain bread (for French toast). Top a sliced banana with pure maple syrup and/or cinnamon. Preparing quick food combinations are not a top priority with kids (although it can be helpful, particularly for kids with tummy aches or digestive issues). See the recipes for the Simple Detox Pizza (page 136) and Detox Quesadilla (page 137), which kids *love*. Make nachos by melting cheddar-style raw goat cheese over Guiltless Gourmet brand chips, topping them with some fresh salsa. Use the same cheese on sprouted grain bread and bake for delicious cheese melts. The options are as endless as your children's appetites.

### Sample Children's Menu

(Italicized recipes are in this book)

**Upon rising:** 1 large glass freshly extracted fruit or vegetable juice (if they are old enough, let them make it—it can be fun!)

**Breakfast Options (choose one or two)**

- 1 large bowl fresh fruit, fresh fruit juice, or fresh raw smoothie.

- 1 bowl Health Valley cereal with a drizzle of honey and Pacific almond milk.

- Sprouted grain bagel with organic butter.

- Raw granola (try Lydia's Grainless Granola) with almond milk and pure maple syrup.

- Homemade French toast: use the sprouted grain bread and whole organic eggs. Top with 100-percent pure maple syrup or agave nectar, cinnamon, and nutmeg.

- Homemade pancakes: make a batter using spelt or kamut flour, whole organic eggs, and almond milk. Top with 100-percent pure maple syrup or agave nectar, cinnamon, and nutmeg.

- Sprouted grain toast with goat yogurt (fruit on the bottom is okay if sugarless).

- Organic free-range eggs, any style—you may use a pat of organic butter to cook and/or add some goat cheese for a yummy cheese omelet.

**Mid-morning snack:** Any fresh raw fruit (grapes, sectioned oranges, apples, and bananas are easy to pack); celery with raw almond butter; dried (unsulfured) fruit like figs or apples, with or without raw nuts. Health Valley also makes some delicious cereal bars that you can include once or twice a week. The raw treats are great at this time, too!

**Lunch Options (choose one)**

- Cheddar-style goat cheese with mustard, tomato, lettuce, and sprouts (optional) on sprouted bread

- Raw almond butter and honey on sprouted grain bread

- Sprouted grain tortilla wraps filled with hummus-covered veggies, or veggies with avocado and salsa

- An Avocado-Vegetable Sandwich on sprouted grain bread

- Crunchy raw salad with organic chicken slices

Ideally, your children would not drink any processed drinks. However, you could include a travel-sized rice milk or chocolate rice milk in their lunch. There are also some great Olive Oil brand sweet potato chips on the market and delicious cookies by Santa Fe Farms that are a great alternative to regular cookies.

**Snack Options**
- Fresh, raw fruits or vegetable (precut watermelon cubes, washed grapes, and peeled carrots with a great raw dip)

- Dried fruits (raisins, apricots, figs, and so forth)

- Raw nuts (macadamias, walnuts, pistachios, and so forth)

- Raw treats (raw packaged foods)

- Lara bars

- Organic vegan bars

- Young coconuts

- Alta Dena raw cheddar-style goat cheese slices with Ak-Mak crackers

- Air-popped popcorn

- Kamut or spelt cakes by Suzie's

- Guiltless Gourmet chips

- Fruit leathers

- Fresh smoothies and shakes

**Dinner Options:** Have a sit-down family dinner as often as possible. Always start the meal with a large raw salad and a delicious raw dressing. Raw sliced beets, jicama, carrots, snow peas, and raw corn, are some good salad ingredients. (Don't use broccoli, cauliflower, or other vegetables that are unpalatable when raw. This will only put your kids off.) After the salad course, enjoy any properly combined meal of your choice including:

- Whole-wheat pasta with Seeds of Change sauce

- Brown rice with organic butter and steamed vegetables

- Grilled fish or baked/grilled/rotisserie chicken with vegetables

- Sweet potatoes or mashed sweet potatoes and vegetables

- Kamut pasta with the cheddar-style goat cheese and sea salt—it's like mac 'n cheese!

- *Detox Pizza*

- *Detox Quesadilla*

- Any high-quality vegetable based soup or a Taste Adventure brand soup

- Any high-quality food your family likes, even if it's a typical breakfast food

**Dessert Options:** Remember you can use raw honey, pure maple syrup, stevia or Splenda, agave nectar, dates or other dried fruits to sweeten dessert. You can also easily achieve fatty tastes and textures by using nut butters, avocados, and coconuts. Desserts can be an "every meal" affair when you're using these high-quality ingredients. That will have your kids coming back for more! Here are just a few ideas:

- A regular or frozen banana drenched in *You-Must-be-Kidding Chocolate Sauce*

- ½ Goldie's carob bar

- 1 scoop Rice Dream ice cream

- Kollar cookies with a glass of almond milk

- Sesame and honey candy

- *Hot Chocolate* with a favorite raw treat

- *Raw Ice Cream* topped with *You-Must-be-Kidding Chocolate Sauce* and nuts (add bananas for a raw-nana split!)

- Raw pie like *Raw Cinnamon Apple-Pear Pie*

**Beverages**
- Carrot juice

- *Green Lemonade*

- Coconut water

- Organic apple juice (preferably raw cider)

- Unpasteurized orange juice

- Almond milk

- Water with a squeeze of lemon or lime and a packet of stevia—what I call a "quick lemonade!"

The trick for busy parents is to get your child involved with the preparation of these meals. Get them acquainted with how to use and clean the juicer. It's really fun to make juices together. When I was a child, my mother used to call them "cocktails." We had such fun making and drinking all the different colored elixirs—thanks Mom!

The other trick is presentation. You must, at least in the beginning, make these foods look beautiful on the plate. It isn't hard to make colorful raw salads look appealing. I suggest making each plate up in the kitchen, adding fresh herbs like cilantro and basil for older children and your spouse. Let everyone dress their own salad at the table so that the salad is served looking crisp. Let your kids build vegetable faces! You can also put out some raw jicama and carrots for the kids to snack on while you prepare dinner. Kids love crunchy, watery vegetables!

According to a report by The Better Health Channel, "Overweight or obese children are more likely to remain obese as adolescents than slimmer children. Adolescence appears to be a particularly sensitive period for the development of obesity. About 80 percent of obese adolescents will become obese adults. Obese children are also more likely to:

- Not do well academically

- Have poor job prospects

- Be socially isolated

Research shows that obese children feel that being overweight is a worse disability than losing a limb."

Children simply should not have to suffer from this kind of "disability." Learning from parents about food and how to eat well is truly invaluable.

# PREGNANCY AND NURSING

Pregnancy and nursing are sacred times for a mother and her baby. For many women, pregnancies result in what appears to be permanent extra weight, leading to terrible frustration and contributing to postpartum depression. But this doesn't have to be the case! There is no reason why you should resign yourself to a matronly figure that's several sizes larger than your prepregnancy figure! A properly executed pregnancy diet can not only help create a perfect, vibrant baby, but it can keep you looking like a "babe" during and after pregnancy!

Whether you're twenty-six or forty-six, you can have a healthy, strong, and yes, *lean* natal and postnatal body by following a gradual transition detox diet between Levels 3 to 5. (If you started out as a Level 1 or 2, you can continue at that level as long as it feels comfortable for you.) The Raw Food Detox Diet is rich in all the nutrients that you and your growing baby need—including the organic forms of these vitamins and minerals, which is essential for maximum absorption.

Pregnant women not only need adequate nutrition but also foods that generate increased energy. It is crucial for the health of a growing baby that the mother eat a diet made up predominantly of organic fruits and vegetables. However, typical pregnancy diets underplay the importance of raw plant food and overemphasize the need for animal products, particularly dairy. Now that you know how dairy and high-protein diets can leach calcium from your body (and keep it from reaching your baby), it's easy to see why a mother's need for plant food increases substantially during pregnancy and nursing.

What I appreciated most about following the program during both my pregnancies was that I experienced very little digestive discomfort. During pregnancy, digestion slows, creating a prime breeding ground for excess gas, bloating, and painful heartburn. But by properly combining my meals, I was able to facilitate digestion and avoid those uncomfortable symptoms; I slept better, had more energy, and—best of all—avoided having to take Tums (which only adds more sugar and inorganic calcium to the body)!

One critical thing to keep in mind, if you're embarking on this diet during your pregnancy, is not to focus on detoxification. If you're accustomed to the standard American diet, pregnancy is *not* the time suddenly to become a raw-food vegan; the toxins that will move through your blood and lymph fluid will cross the placenta and likely affect your baby. Instead, focus on quick exit food combinations and aim for a 50 to 60 percent raw diet, which you can consistently—but slowly—increase if you're comfortable throughout your pregnancy. This is one time when you should definitely continue to eat small amounts of flesh and dairy to avoid triggering too many detoxifying symptoms all at once. You'll do very well and avoid excess weight gain just by properly combining foods and eating your fruits and greens. Once the baby is born and you start nursing, you may increase your raw foods and eliminate the flesh foods, if you're ready. Then, if you commit to the Raw Food Detox Diet steps in this book, you will eventually get back to your leanest and most vibrant self!

## Sample Raw Food Detox Diet Pregnancy Regimen

Suggested Prenatal Daily Intake

> **Upon rising:** 12 to 16 ounces of freshly extracted green juice with an apple added for sweetness. (You may add garlic and ginger, but they can be very off-putting early on in pregnancy.) The leafy greens will provide the organic calcium and folic acid you need for the baby and to protect your own calcium stores (which can be drained and hard to replace in later years) during pregnancy. Spinach is the most valuable of the leafy vegetables, as it is more than 88-percent water and has the finest quality of obtainable organic iron.
>
> **Breakfast:** Any fruit of your choice (just remember to eat melons before other fruit, as they digest more quickly)

Whenever you feel the need for a heartier breakfast (or starchy food in the morning during the early months of pregnancy), you may have any hot or cold whole grain, naturally sweetened cereal of your choice with almond milk. You may use raw honey to sweeten your cereal, if desired. Raw sprouted grains and soaked nuts with raw honey and almond milk offer a powerful fat-protein, antioxidant, zinc-rich punch!

Alternatively, you may have toasted sprouted grain bread, sprouted grain bagels, or whole wheat pita with real organic butter. But digestion and energy will be best when you only consume fresh fruit or the "Smooth Mamma" shake (see below) in the morning after your green juice.

> **Mid-morning snack:** Smooth Mama shake: 2 to 3 teaspoons of Sun Chlorella blended into a smoothie of 1 banana, a splash of freshly squeezed juice or water, and 2 to 3 tablespoons of raw walnuts. While the shake will look very green, it will actually taste very sweet.
>
> **Lunch:** You may enjoy any of the dishes from the recipe section depending on your level of the program, accompanied by raw vegetables or a raw vegetable salad.
>
> **Mid-afternoon snack:** This is an ideal time to have another fresh veggie juice or a "Smooth Mama." Drink it on an empty stomach. If you're still hungry, you may

follow this drink thirty minutes later with 2 stalks of celery with raw almond butter and honey, dried fruit, fresh fruit, fresh fruit juice, or a handful of raw nuts of your choice. Almonds and walnuts are ideal. Pecans back a terrific zinc punch, as do Brazil nuts and pistachios; your zinc needs to increase during pregnancy.

**Dinner:** You may have any of the dishes in this book's recipe section or restaurant section. Just be sure to include a raw salad.

**Dessert:** Several squares of carob, pure chocolate, or a whole grain cookie. Pregnant women run the risk of hypertension and high blood pressure, for which raw garlic can be highly beneficial. This is another great reason for discontinuing the consumption of coffee, sodas, and other caffeinated substances.

Most new mothers have heard that protein and calcium are very important during pregnancy. However, it is not necessary to consume large amounts of animal products to achieve these nutritional requirements. In fact, animal protein can leach calcium from the body and is very difficult for the body to break down, making it more difficult to utilize than plant protein—not to mention all the antibiotics, hormones, parasites, and other pollutants that you find in animal protein. This is not to say that you cannot enjoy an omnivorous diet during your pregnancy; just know that eating animal protein is not necessary to nurture your body and your growing baby.

The most digestible, effective protein and calcium for the body comes from raw plant foods and nature's "superfoods"—chlorella (65 percent assimilable protein/5 grams of protein per teaspoon/15 grams of protein per tablespoon) and bee pollen.

## Pregnancy Tips

■ Eat plenty of fresh fruit in the morning to stay hydrated, get the necessary sugars without feeling heavy, and prevent water retention. All that hydration will mean you won't have to drink so much water.

■ If nothing else, stick to quick exit food combinations. That alone will keep your system moving smoothly, ensure maximum intake of nutrients, and prevent excess weight gain.

■ If you are eating according to the Raw Food Detox Diet principles, don't worry if you put on 40 pounds during your pregnancy. Every woman and every baby are different. If you gain 40 pounds on this program while pregnant, that's what you and your body need, and it will come off swiftly.

- When you crave something starchy, enjoy the sprouted grain breads, sweet potatoes, and spelt cakes.

- Once you have had your baby, your weight should come off within four to five months. If, after six months postpartum you are still struggling with your last 10 pounds, simply undertake a short juice fast (see page 227). By this point, you can safely do this while nursing. Six months after each of my pregnancies, I did a six-day juice fast and had tons of rich milk for my babies. I also whittled myself into my best shape ever!

### Is it safe to undertake this program while nursing?

Nursing on this program is like entering The Land of Milk and Honey: You will produce superior quality milk for your baby while achieving your best body ever. There is nothing more magical, natural, and fulfilling than nursing your baby. The time you spend with him or her in those quite hours will enrich both of you in immeasurable ways that will last a lifetime. Unfortunately, many mothers give up on nursing prematurely. Here are the five main reasons why:

1. The mother doesn't realize how much of a time commitment nursing requires.

2. The pediatrician recommends formula supplementation before the mother has a chance to establish her milk supply, so she fears that her milk is inadequate for her baby's development.

3. The mother's nutrient intake is insufficient for a rich, satisfying milk supply.

4. The baby doesn't get enough sucking time at the breast.

5. The mother employs a breast pump before her milk supply becomes well established.

Let's address each issue individually:

### Nursing Nemesis #1: The mother doesn't realize how much of a time commitment nursing requires.

No one tells you the really important things about motherhood and nursing. A new mother with the ambition to breastfeed is hardly ever told that for the first six to eight weeks, to nurse successfully long term, she will have to fully commit herself to breastfeeding her child as though it is her full-time job. She must be prepared to spend the first two months of new motherhood nursing her baby on demand.

When I first started breastfeeding my daughter, I got myself a little notebook in which I daily recorded each feeding time—in the hopes that I would be able to develop a pattern that I could stick to with each consecutive day. Well, as it turned out, my little notebook's pages were too small to hold the long list of feeding times, which looked something like this: 7:30 A.M., 8:45 A.M., 10:00 A.M., 12:00 P.M., 12:45 P.M., 2:00 P.M., 4:30 P.M., 5:00 P.M., 6:45 P.M., 8:00 P.M., 8:50 P.M., 11:00 P.M., 1:00 A.M., 2:45 A.M., 5:00 A.M. . . . and on and on it went.

The first few days, I was averaging twelve feedings a day! That is not at all what I envisioned when I dreamed of nursing my baby. And yes, I had read all the books on the subject. To make matters worse, those books left me with the impression that I was failing my daughter somehow if I didn't keep her to a strict three-hour feeding schedule (which wasn't her natural schedule at all in the early weeks) All the while, she seemed to cry endlessly every time I removed her from the breast.

## Nursing Nemesis #2: The pediatrician recommends formula supplementation before the mother has a chance to establish her milk supply, so she fears that her milk is inadequate for her baby's development.

After five weeks of trying frantically to get life back to normal while nursing, the pediatrician recommended that I start to feed my daughter formula, as she wasn't putting on weight fast enough. So, in addition to feeling that I'd failed at creating a schedule, I was told was that my milk wasn't even properly nourishing my baby!

Wanting to do the right thing for my five-week-old girl, I went to the supermarket to purchase baby formula—even though I considered it poison. Every time I fed her the formula, I felt worse about it. Her lovely baby smell turned into that terrible formula smell, and she started to spit up for the first time. I figured that there had to be another way, so I set out to find it. Two weeks after beginning formula, I threw it out and put my research to work for my daughter. I was determined to give her the high-quality precious milk she deserved—mine!

## Nursing Nemesis #3: The mother's nutrient intake is insufficient for a rich, satisfying milk supply.

The second step was to radically change my diet. While I had been sticking to a 75-percent raw diet with proper food combinations during pregnancy, the lactation therapists at the hospital told me that to make milk I would need to eat things like steak, ice-cream, milk, potatoes, and other high-calorie foods. But then it occurred to me that cows don't drink milk or eat meat to make milk. In fact, they eat grass. So I decided to start eating like a cow! Needing calcium-rich greens to make abundant milk, I started consuming 2 pounds of greens each day. I ate 1 pound in its raw form (lettuce, mesclun, spinach, and so forth) and 1 pound steamed (broccoli, chard, asparagus, and so forth). I had let my milk supply diminish for nearly two weeks, so I had to go to extremes to get it flowing again.

In addition to these two crucial changes, I started to incorporate the more natural essential fatty acids and omega-3's (essential for infants' brain development): avocados, walnuts, tahini, and some salmon. Within one week, I was feeding Thandi exclusively on breast milk again. She was happy, and I was thrilled. After a few weeks, Thandi gradually started feeding at two and three hour intervals, and with each week the nursing became easier and easier.

## Nursing Nemesis #4: The baby doesn't get enough sucking time at the breast.

The first thing I did was commit to nursing my daughter as often and as long as she would let me. I learned that the more a baby sucks, the more milk there will be the following day. The reason Thandi had cried so much initially was because she needed the closeness of being nursed *and* she had the biological need to suckle in order to signal to my breasts just how much milk she would need the next day! If I had realized from the get-go that I was going to need to nurse so much, I would have prepared myself for that and wouldn't have become so stressed.

## Nursing Nemesis #5: The mother employs a breast pump before her milk supply becomes well established.

Breast pumps are a must-have for just about every nursing mother in the western world. However, if used too early (except in the case of premature babies), they can interfere with a mother's milk supply. For example, if a mother starts to pump in the weeks just following her baby's birth because she wants to have milk to bottle and store for her baby (a perfectly natural desire), it may take her ten to fifteen minutes to empty her breasts. But if given the opportunity, the baby would not only empty her mother's breasts but would likely continue to suckle for an additional fifteen to thirty minutes—sending the message that she needs to produce a lot more milk. A mother who bottle-feeds her baby will have less milk the following day than if she had nursed. Using the breast pump once or twice isn't a big deal, but don't let it become a way to avoid your baby's rigorous nursing schedule.

Once your milk supply is fully established (only after ten to twelve weeks of giving birth), you can begin to use your pump regularly. But try to avoid doing so (except on the odd occasion) before that time, as you don't want to upset nature's superior milk-response system.

### Additional Nursing Tips

1. Eat at least 5 servings of fresh, raw fruit daily (best on an empty stomach in the morning, or at least three hours after a properly combined meal).

2. Consume large amounts of green vegetables daily. Try to consume at least ½ pound raw green leafy vegetables. The rest can be lightly steamed or sautéed. I also recommend drinking 20 ounces of freshly extracted green juice (with apple for sweetness).

3. Consume essential fatty acids (EFA's) and omega-3's daily. You can do this by taking 2 tablespoons of Udo's Oil (a flax oil blend) daily and eating avocados and raw nuts (walnuts are very high in EFAs). While fatty fish is also a good source, there are many potentially harmful pollutants in fish today, so do not eat too much fish.

4. Nursing on demand as often as possible in the first six to eight weeks will ensure a lasting and abundant milk supply. Avoid pumping until you've established your milk supply. If you want to go out for a few hours but worry about your baby going hungry, try diluting goat milk—1 part goat milk to 2 parts water—as a substitute for breast milk from the very first week. (Remember to first check with your baby's pediatrician.)

### What's the difference between breast milk and formula from a physiological standpoint?

The decision to breastfeed your infant is one that will stay with your child long after the first year or two of life. The American Academy of Pediatrics recommends breast milk for the first year of life and documents numerous breast-feeding advantages for the newborn:

- Increase in IQ scores later in childhood

- Enhanced neurodevelopmental performance

■ Lower incidence of the following conditions: allergies and asthma, bacteremia and meningitis, childhood lymphoma, chronic constipation, diabetes, gastrointestinal infections, infantile eczema, inflammatory bowel disease, iron deficiency anemia, lower respiratory tract infections, sudden infant death syndrome, urinary tract infections

Despite the fact that pediatricians put their stamp of approval on commercial formulas, there simply is no substitute for breast milk. Perhaps the most important difference between formula and breast milk is the effect that the latter has on brain development. Breast milk contains long-chain polyunsaturated fatty acids such as docosahexaenoic acid (DHA) and arachidonic acid (AA), which are essential for brain development.

Additionally, there is a neurobiological mechanism in normal growth and development involving tryptophane—a precursor amino acid essential for the development of brain serotonin, which is richly present in colostrum and breast milk but absent in formula milk. This mechanism has been proven critical to successful human development. Without tryptophane and the physical, sensory bonding of the mother-infant relationship, an infant won't be able to develop optimal levels of serotonin and will be robbed of enhanced cognitive development.

It is even more critical for a premature child to receive mother's milk. And it just so happens that the milk produced by a mother of a preterm infant is higher in protein and other nutrients than that of the mother of a full-term infant. This precious preterm milk will also protect the preemie against infections, offering the child the immunity that his/her own little body has not yet developed.

There are four of the key building blocks of infant nutrition: selenium, an antioxidant and mineral that plays a key role in balancing nutrition; nucleotides, the bulding blocks of genetic material; beta-carotene, immune and tissue support; and LCPs, long-chain polyunsaturated fatty acids essential for vision, nervous system, and brain development. All of these are found naturally in breast milk. Breast milk offers greater protection against iron deficiency anemia than cow's milk or a non-iron-fortified formula. While the iron content of breast milk is lower than that of cow's milk, it is about five times better absorbed—due in part to its high lactose and vitamin C content. The large quantity of lactose in breast milk contributes to the development of the central nervous system and the intestinal flora. Also note that an infant can use 100 percent of the protein in breast milk, but only 50 percent of the protein in cow's milk.

Not only will your *baby* thrive on the milk that this Raw Food Detox Diet for pregnancy produces, but *you* will also attain the best shape of your life. Breastfeeding will help make both of you vibrant and healthy—and is quite possibly a mother's best tool in raising a truly joyful child.

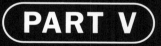

# PART V

# THE ASPIRING RAW FOODIST

# RAW DONE RIGHT

Take off all your clothes and stand in front of the mirror. Now look at your midsection, your eyes, your ankles, your facial tone, your hips. Do you look like pristine man or woman? Now take a look inside: what is your emotional and psychological state—are you even-tempered, calm, joyful, and harmonious (without the help of pharmaceutical or recreational drugs)? Can you easily skip a couple of meals and feel perfectly calm?

If you've answered "yes" to these questions, then you're free to become a raw foodist overnight. You have my blessing. If, however, you answered "no" to any of these questions, then you'll want to take a slightly different approach to the powerful raw elements. I like to call it "progress through transition," and it is fundamental to the Raw Food Detox Diet. In other words, it is not necessary or even advisable to tackle a 100-percent raw food diet to take your cellular health and physique to peak condition. In fact, by keeping some cooked foods in your diet, you will progress faster than a prematurely plunged 100-percent raw food dieter. Here's why.

As you know, raw foods (plant foods not heated above 118°F) contain life force energy from the sun. This life force energy is very powerful and can help the body heal itself. The live enzymes within raw foods serve as catalysts to support every human function. Because your stores of enzymes run dangerously low in adulthood (after years of eating enzyme-less foods), a sudden influx of live enzymes can enable your body to return to its higher functioning condition of youth. This is one way you use raw foods to make you feel younger. In addition to these healing duties, live enzymes also pull out the garbage from your cells for removal. On one hand, this is a very exciting function because it means that years of bad eating and hard living can be reversed. On the other hand, it means that this garbage, when pulled out of your cells, is suddenly somewhere else in your body—namely, in your bloodstream and eliminative organs.

If you transition carefully, by slowly increasing your intake of raw foods, and ensure that that garbage is fully eliminated through increased bowel activity, sweat, deep breathing, massage, and adequate, gentle sunlight, you will gracefully and easily turn over a new body. However (and this is a big "however"), if you decide one morning to "go all raw," all that garbage is going to hit a major traffic jam, which will culminate in gassiness, constipation, skin eruptions, and fatigue. All that garbage you worked so hard to draw up by eating only raw foods is not exiting your body, so it's back to the bloodstream for those toxins, and you never get beyond your old cellular condition. Raw foods are incredibly powerful—they stir things up! Just remember, while they can dislodge impaction in the body from as far back as your childhood, you don't want to misuse them.

Although a 100-percent raw food diet would certainly be ideal for humans living in a 100-percent natural state, we live in a world riddled with unnatural elements. For modern people like us, there is a safe way to carry our tissue/cell quality to a much higher level with raw foods. But we must do it within the context of who and where we are today.

Now let's get back to the body that stands before you in the mirror. It is asking you to appreciate its unique need for a gentle transition. Taking this approach to becoming a raw foodist will bring you far more success than a worthless label. You will gain the confidence of perfect health and a renewed, glowing body.

# RAW LABELS DO NOT MAKE YOU HEALTHY

People too often feel the need to label the way they are eating. Aspiring raw foodists are no different. But a label has never made anyone healthy. The trick to eating this way long-term is to avoid feeling bound to a diet label. Sure, you might feel very strongly about eating exclusively raw—right now. But what happens when you find yourself feeling bored and lacking imagination in the kitchen or going to your favorite restaurant and craving some jumbo curried shrimp? Then what? I'll tell you what: go ahead and have that jumbo curried shrimp and enjoy it. Occasionally treating yourself to your favorite dinner meal (provided it's well-combined) will make you feel all the more satisfied with your approach to raw foods.

This is why I recommend including the raw cheddar-style goat cheese as a staple of your diet. This cheese is highly satisfying and, as long as you don't eat it all the time, it won't interfere with your progress. It's important to remind yourself how well you can eat while cultivating a cleaner, healthier body. When you limit yourself, you shut down your natural desires, whereas this program is about *enhancing* your natural desires. Your desires will change tremendously when you undertake the cleansing process, and you'll be able to trust them more because you'll undoubtedly be craving high-quality foods. If you open yourself up to many tastes and flavors, nonvegan and nonraw foods among them, you will have greater success in the long run—I promise!

During the years that I was transitioning to "all raw," I struggled with what to call myself. I wasn't officially a "raw foodist" since I still ate some cooked food. Even though I wasn't eating more than a couple of cooked meals a week, it simply seemed untruthful to call myself a raw foodist. I wasn't vegan or vegetarian either because at least one of those cooked meals that I'd eat each week included fish. The term that I came up with was "aspiring raw foodist," and it felt right for a while. But then I realized that the term could easily be misconstrued, depending on the connotation it carried for different people. Some raw foodists are wise and loving, whereas others are militant and judgmental. Why in the world would I attach myself to a label that does not necessarily represent me? So I decided that I wouldn't. From that day forward, I would say, "No labels, thank you very much! I eat what I eat when I want to, and that's that." How incredibly liberating!

# TRANSITION—DON'T DIVE HEAD FIRST INTO THE DEEP END OF THE RAW FOOD POOL

As you've learned, it is critical to find your proper Raw Food Transition Number and stick with it until your body agrees that you are ready to move on. Don't sabotage your health by forcing yourself too eat too healthfully—an ironic statement, perhaps, but one that I base on years of experience. Listen to your cleansing symptoms (such as heavy-headedness, sluggishness, moodiness, acne, and so forth) that show your bowel is not keeping pace with waste that's being stirred up. Support your body's rejuvenating efforts by maintaining an intimate dialogue with it. Anyone who is into health for the right reasons shouldn't intimidate or manipulate you into eating all raw with dogma—least of all, yourself!

# KEEP THE GOAL IN MIND

Your goal is superior cell health, not an exclusively raw food diet. Raw is a means of reaching that goal. The goal of being 100-percent raw is like being 100-percent focused on your work instead of your life as a whole. Work is not the goal; a happy, balanced, successful life is the goal. If you become exclusively focused on work, you will miss out on the best parts of your life.

To achieve the goal of superior cell health (i.e., a younger feeling, leaner you), you need enzymes from raw foods, maximum elimination of the waste matter those enzymes draw up, and tempered amounts of cooked foods—to avoid autointoxication and keep your emotional, social, and physiological states intact.

# GREENS AND GREEN LEMONADE ARE YOUR RAW CURRENCY

You cannot detoxify successfully without committing to a steady intake of green vegetable juice. Green vegetable juice is the lifeblood of a successful raw food diet. The abundance of chlorophyll, organic minerals, and enzymes in the juice will neutralize your body's acidy with its rich alkalinity. Green is the color of healing, signifying the way plants synthesize sunlight into the life force that is essential to our health. In fact, the chlorophyll molecule is similarly structured to the hemin molecule of hemoglobin (blood). In addition to sending freshly oxygenated living cells into the bloodstream to recharge our blood, the chlorophyll works as an excellent blood builder; whereas hemin has iron as it's central atom, chlorophyll has magnesium. It's okay if you miss your green vegetable juice for a day or two, but do make it a staple of your diet.

# DON'T BE DENSE

Dense raw foods are just as clogging as many cooked foods. One of the biggest mistakes in the popular raw food movement is trying to mimic mainstream diets with raw food substitutes. This is very similar to what happened when vegetarianism took hold in the 70s. Suddenly vegetarians were eating burgers, fish patties, and eggs made out of tofu and other heavily processed plant foods. The point of eating raw foods is to eat light foods—not, for instance, to create a heavy loaf out of nuts. You may as well be eating a meat loaf as far as your digestive system is concerned! On the Raw Food Detox Diet, you can eat raw most of the time, but when you want, say, a piece of fish, you can eat a piece of fish—not a dense, sprouted, dehydrated "unfish."

The emotional satisfaction that you will get from occasionally eating a familiar, nonraw dish will keep the raw foods fun. The whole psychology of "forbidden fruit" is too much of a burden for most people, and it's unnecessary for this way of eating. Forget the dogma; for health and weight loss, you are far better off choosing a fish and vegetable dinner over a dense, nut-based raw meal.

# FOCUS BEFORE YOU FAST

Fasting could not have a better, more concise definition than "nature's operating table." When you fast, you shut down digestion so that all of your energy can go toward healing your body at every level (your cells, tissues, and organs). Thus, you are literally placing yourself in the hands of the most adept surgeon there is: nature. Your body is designed to heal itself, but is not often given the opportunity to do so because you're constantly forcing it to spend its healing energy on managing external factors such as food, pollution, stress, excessive exercise, and so forth.

You might compare nature's healing method to that of an emergency room complete with a triage system. The triage system sends help to the places in the body where the most energy is required at the time. Once help arrives, the body goes to work on that area of the body. This system is a tremendous gift, a glimpse into natural law (the laws of nature that govern our physicality) at work. However, the typical western diet and lifestyle abuses this gift by creating so many burdens on the body each day that this system cannot possibly get help to all of the areas in need. Imagine an emergency room filled with so many injured patients that, by the end of the day, only half of them have received the attention they need. This is exactly what is happening within your body on a daily basis. The most obvious offender of this system happens to be your diet.

Through the Raw Food Detox Diet, you can clear up the backlog that is created by years of eating poor food and poor food combinations. By fasting, you can occasionally give your body a complete break from digestion so that it can heal even more deeply.

However, just because fasting is a highly effective method of detoxifying more deeply, it's not necessary at every stage. You needn't even consider fasting unless (1) you have a distinct desire to do so—whether for personal, spiritual, or physical reasons; (2) you have hit a wall in the cleansing progress and you want a great way to break through that wall.

There are many different kinds of fasts—water fasts, juice fasts, blended food fasts—on which you only consume a particular substance. While there are many popular methods of fasting, there is only one way to infuse your body with enzymes, vitamins, minerals, and organic water while completely resting the digestive track. This method is "juice fasting," and it is the most effective, pleasant, and safe way to fast.

Those of you who have never fasted before might doubt your ability to go without food much longer than the typical nine to twelve hours between dinner and breakfast. Before actually experiencing the pleasures of a fast, the term can connote a bleak, dull, lonely experience. You can probably hear the grumbling of your tummy just thinking of it. But ask people who have juice-fasted to boost their health, and they'll tell you that the time they spent consuming only fresh, raw juices, herbal teas, and vegetable broth was invigorating and transforming—both physically and psychologically.

Something wonderful happens to every aspect of your being when you take several days to rest your digestive system. Taking a break from food for a reasonable period of time can have a radically positive effect on your internal cleansing system. It enables your body to dramatically rid itself of excess waste in your cells, like no other method of dieting can. You may have noticed that animals instinctively fast when they are sick, just as children tend to lose their appetite when they are ill. Fasting is a natural phenomenon.

However, how you choose to fast is critical. You must take the time to plan for a good fast. In fact, you must have a pre-fast eating plan—know which juices you will fast on and how you'll be encouraging the body to eliminate the toxins that will be stirred up. And, most importantly, you need to know how to break the fast.

Let's start with the pre-fast menu. During the two to three days before you fast, it is best to avoid all unnatural foods and animal products. While it's not mandatory, it will make for a less severe transition. During a fast, you will want to employ as many of the "waste management specialists" (i.e., colonics, sweating, body brushing, and so forth) as possible. Resting is a good idea, but not essential. On a juice fast, you should have plenty of energy. Unlike water-fasting, you will be getting natural sugars, enzymes, vitamins, and minerals into your bloodstream, so you should feel as strong as ever. You may get a bit "racy" or feel "high" after a couple of days of fasting, but this is a great feeling to look forward to. I consider it an incredible lightness of being—spiritually, emotionally, and physically.

# HOW TO USE FASTING AS A TUNE-UP EVERY FIVE MONTHS

One issue that fasting brings up for many of my clients is their social schedule. They often say that they would love to fast, but they've got to do such and such this week and such and such that week. I will tell you what I tell them: if you really want to fast, you will find a way to set aside a week for it. Those engagements will always be there. Friends will understand. You must decide what is important to you, and then do it.

The other thing that my clients typically say is, "I really want to fast but my family and friends will freak out if I stop eating. They already think I've gone off the deep end eating this way." Again, I'll tell you what I tell them: if you play by everyone else's rules, you'll never know who you are or what you're capable of. The Raw Food Detox Diet is more than just a food lifestyle; it's a mental and spiritual lifestyle as well. Don't let other people's fear of the unknown prevent you from learning and making real progress.

## A Sample Fasting Regimen

1. Early on the first morning of the fast, give yourself a thorough dry body brushing, from the soles of your feet all the way up to the back of your neck.

2. After the body brushing, you may drink tea or hot water with lemon juice, or just several glasses of spring or steam-distilled water.

3. An hour or two later, you may take an enema or, ideally, have a colonic.

4. Mid-morning, have your first glass of unpasteurized, freshly extracted fruit juice. If you are using a very sweet fruit like grape or apple, dilute it with water. (If you are juicing a melon or pineapple, juice the rind as well, as it is full of chlorophyll.)

5. Spend the day doing something you really enjoy. You might read a great book, work on a project, organize your home, indulge yourself with a long bath with essential oils, or schedule a massage.

6. Mid-afternoon, take a break from whatever you're doing to enjoy a glass of freshly extracted vegetable juice.

7. Continue working on your chosen project, go for a long walk, meditate, or do yoga.

8. Rest for at least an hour. Take a cup of herbal tea to enjoy at your beside.

9. Take a bath, steam bath, or sauna, followed by a shower.

10. Enjoy another glass of your favorite freshly extracted fruit or vegetable juice.

11. At dinnertime, go for a walk so that you don't feel deprived. When you return, give yourself another dry body brushing, enjoy more herbal tea, and settle in for an early, excellent night's sleep. Keep a journal by your bed, as you'll likely have revelatory dreams!

After two to three days, if that's enough for you, you may begin to break the fast by eating small amounts of raw vegetables. If you have diligently adhered to the Raw Food Detox Diet for several months (without eating large amounts of animal flesh or taking medications) you may break your fast with fresh fruits. You want your first meal after a fast to have a laxative effect—or stimulate your bowels to move. You should have a movement within a couple of hours of eating. The key to breaking any fast is not to overeat. Doing so can undermine all the good that you've accomplished by fasting. In the two days after the fast, you should follow the pre-fast menu of mainly raw fruits and raw or steamed vegetables. Thereafter, go back to eating according to your Raw Food Detox Diet transition level.

A note about preparing for pregnancy: while it is not recommended to fast (even juice fast) while pregnant, juice-fasting is an ideal way to prepare your body for a healthy pregnancy—*before* you get pregnant. Fasting enables the body to eliminate heavy metals and other environmental pollutants that can negatively affect both your fertility and your baby-to-be. (For more information on pregnancy, please see page 208.)

Fasting is not only a way to jump-start weight loss, detoxification, and remedy myriad physical ailments, but also enables you to tap into blocked creative energies and see your life more clearly. Don't let the fear of the unknown prevent you from trying this age-old method of regeneration!

# FREQUENTLY ASKED QUESTIONS ABOUT FASTING

### How long should I fast?

There is great value in mini-fasts. You could start by occasionally juicing until dinner. This helps your body get over the stimulation of food, and is an easy, nonintimidating way to try fasting.

Two to three days is a perfectly good length of time for your first real fast. Thereafter, you can try gradually going a bit longer with each fast, up to a maximum of eight to ten days (unless you are under the guidance of a doctor, a fasting specialist, or colon specialist).

Please note that it's not advisable to fast without some sort of effective bowel release. Remember, the goal of fasting is to rest the body enough to let it draw up old matter. If this matter is not exiting the body, fasting is useless and can even be harmful.

You can also achieve a lot without going on a hard-core juice fast, simply by eating according to natural law, as your body is designed to eat. Like fasting, this way of eating gives the digestive system the rest it needs to begin the deep-tissue healing that's so integral to your health.

### How much weight will I lose on a fast?

You will probably lose about a pound a day. Men may lose more.

### Won't fasting slow down my metabolism, and won't I just regain that weight when I start eating normally again?

No one gains weight simply because the metabolism slows down (as you've learned, your body becomes sluggish when there is too much waste in your cells). It's just that a cleaner body requires less heavy food, so if you go back to eating the same food you ate before making the transition to raw foods, you'll put on weight again. You'll be able to eat the equivalent number of calories from whole, natural foods and keep the weight off because you'll be keeping the *waste* off. So it's not a calorie/metabolism equation. When you fast in conjunction with the elimination of waste, all the excessive weight that comes off will remain off.

### Tips for Successful Fasting

- Plan fun, nonfood activities: go to movies, visit bookstores, go for walks, window-shop, clean out your home, work on a project, and so forth.

- Fast with a friend so you can motivate each other to stick with it, as well as do fun, nonfood activities together. Plan to meet or talk at least once a day. Shop for vegetables and make your juice together.

- Enjoy a day at the spa. Nothing will take your mind off food like a good massage, facial, and haircut.

- Keep a book about fasting with you to read whenever you need a motivational boost.

■ In the evening, take a long bath, go for a walk, or rent a great video. Nighttime is the hardest time for fasting because that's when we look forward to food the most. If you have to cook for others, take pleasure in preparing a meal for them while you sip your juice.

■ Remember, the food is not going anywhere. It will still be there when you're done fasting, and you will be rewarded with a cleaner, leaner, more energetic body.

■ Treat yourself with strained, freshly squeezed orange juice or (on a cold day) hot vegetable broth.

■ Politely ignore comments from well-meaning but uneducated people who criticize you for undertaking a fast. Their comments are probably based on their own fears; people don't always like their friends to change because it threatens their world.

■ Fasting frees up so much time otherwise spent on food preparation. Use that time to get important tasks done. This lifestyle is about freeing up your life and getting to the essentials so that there's time for cultivating your relationships, ambitions, spirituality, and overall happiness!

# FOCUS ON COLON THERAPY

As I mentioned in part I, many of you may choose to enlist the services of a highly-qualified colon therapist to help eliminate the waste matter you'll be dislodging as you incorporate these dietary steps. To further explore the subject and address many of the questions you may have about this alternative therapy, I have interviewed the foremost colon therapist, Gil Jacobs. He also happens to be a highly regarded health counselor and speaker. I have known Gil for many years and refer my clients to him and his partners at his colon health clinic in Manhattan called Chakra 17.

## INTERVIEW WITH MASTER COLON THERAPIST AND CLEANSING GURU, GIL JACOBS

**One of the first concerns people seem to have about colon therapy is that it might cause some structural damage, like rupturing their colon. What would you say to people about this?**

Speaking only to the effects of a gravity centered colonic, which is the only kind of unit I recommend, the water enters the body through a thin tube which has the diameter of approximately ⅙ to ⅛ inch. And if they were to see just how gentle the flow of water is as it enters the body, they would see there is no way anything can be damaged. The water goes through way too slowly and in too small a quantity. You would have to have an intestine that was made of papier-mâché for that water to do any damage whatsoever.

If a gravity centered colonic could create a problem, then enemas could create the same problem because the water from a colonic goes in no more powerfully than the water from an enema. The difference is just that more water goes in over time. No one has ever, ever had a risk of rupturing a bowel with an enema. Hospitals administer enemas regularly and there is not a gastrointestinal doctor in the world who is going to tell you that an enema runs the risk of rupturing or tearing the bowel. A gravity centered colonic follows the exact same principle. It just goes on longer. A colonic is actually far safer because it will remove the water and matter regardless of the sickness or weakness of the individual, whereas an enema relies on the strength of the individual to pass the water and matter out of the bowel. An individual who is sick and overweight won't always be strong enough. What scares people is that a colonic takes forty-five minutes and uses over twenty gallons of water. Hydraulic pressure colonics, on the other hand, are in my estimation dangerous because the water is electrically pushed into the body and then suctioned out, instead of working with gravity and momentum. I don't endorse those.

**The second most common concern is that laxatives and colonics are addictive. How is it that laxatives can be addictive but colonics are not?**

Most people who take laxatives all the time tend to have really bad eating habits, whereas people who get into colonics are doing so from a holistic point of view. We have to remember that *holistic* doesn't mean "natural"; the term comes from *hologram* meaning "whole" or "the entire thing." For the most part, people who get into colonics as part of their life experience—which can mean anything from one colonic a month to one colonic a week—are eating a diet that is high in alkalinity, high in oxygen, and very low in starch, protein, and acid. Ergo, the colonics aid in the flushing out of *old* poison. But because their diet is so good and the food is so easily moved through the body, they never get dependent and they never get to the point where they have to do it all the time.

When we discuss laxatives, we're usually talking about people who are suffering from psychological food disorders, where they are using laxatives to knock out cheeseburgers and French fries. That won't work because this type of food sticks to the intestinal wall like glue. The laxative is an irritant. I love to call it "the mousetrap on the finger of the one armed man." If you put a mousetrap on your finger and you only have one arm, you are going to shake, shake, shake that arm to get the mousetrap off. That's similar to what a laxative does for someone who eats poorly. If you're using laxatives to eliminate normal, heavy, acidic food, you will become dependent because normal, heavy, acidic food is not passable to most human bodies.

The other factor is that the colonic is not a stimulant or an irritant, but a totally different thing altogether. It's the use of water to remove matter. A laxative can only knock out what you put in the body a day or two before, if you're lucky. I'm of the opinion that when people take laxatives and eat lousy, they are not eliminating waste at all; they are just leaking electrolytes. Most people will tell you that laxatives give them the runs. Heavy food, when it leaves the body, is always in a solid state. So, when people get leaky from taking things like citrate and magnesium, the heavy matter that they are trying to get out is sticking to the walls of the colon while all these liquid minerals then roll off the side of it. So a colonic is not addictive to people who are eating the way they are supposed to.

A good therapist coming from a place of integrity would be able to tell if someone is eating mainstream, low-quality, heavy foods when (a) the colonic hurts because the normal foods stick like cement and (b) the colonic doesn't release anything after the initial one or two treatments because of the shock to the body. The initial one or two treatments can work on anyone because the body is so surprised. But after that, if someone were to continue on a regular basis while eating the standard American diet, the treatments will actually release nothing because colonics are in and of themselves useless.

However, people undertaking this raw food lifestyle will have tremendous results with colonics because all the good food (the juice, salads, fruits, and so forth) that they're taking in will awaken the old "demons" and remove them. Adults who have grown up on normal food in their twenties, thirties, fourties [and] convert to a diet that's 80 percent salad, vegetable juice, and fruit and 20 percent that's avocado, nuts, seeds, cooked grains and cooked tubers, could do one colonic a week for life because their bodies are so filled with waste from all the previous years of eating normally.

A laxative on its best day will do nothing for someone who is eating well, except remove matter from the day before. The older, denser matter, very often with laxatives will back up deeper into the tissues and all that will come out is newer matter. So the older matter that the person is attempting to cleanse actually gets more stuck and goes deeper into the tissue. The difference between colonics and laxatives is astronomical. For a person who is eating well, a colonic can remove matter from days gone by. A gravity method colonic will not irritate the body. It will strengthen the body's ability to work on its own because the colonic works with the person's own peristalsis (the natural contractions of the muscular walls of the bowel that move bowel contents forward). A laxative does not work with peristalsis; it just irritates the bowel. So they are two very different things. And again, people who do colonics for the right reasons are already on a very healthful, cleansing diet. If they are not doing colonics for the right reasons, but rather from a psychological food disorder, any therapist with integrity will refuse to treat them.

**What would you tell someone who's reading this book but can't get to a colon therapist?**
Starting bowel-cleansing work is such a new thing for the average young or middle-age adult that, for the initial month that you're eating well, almost anything you do is going to work. You

could take bulb enemas, which are two- or three-ounce infant ear syringes; you could take Fleet enemas (replace the water with fresh water); you could take Swiss Kriss or any herbal laxative. The issue isn't for the beginner. The issue is for the person who gets deep into tissue cleansing when they've been at this for two, three, or four years.

The enema will sometimes tease old, difficult matter that the person doesn't have the capacity to pass on his or her own. At this time, the enema becomes questionable because it will push the matter deeper into the bowel wall while simply removing the lighter matter from the previous twelve hours. This is why many people who do enemas complain of a lot of cloudiness in the head and tightness in the solar plexus. So if you're a beginner who is just reading this and getting into bowel cleansing, Fleet enemas, bulb enemas, and 2-quart bag enemas will work for a while. But if, all of a sudden, they stop working, it's usually because you're getting to some deeper putrified matter.

If you're trying to be 100-percent raw or you're a women who has bowel issues, you might want to invest in a Colema Board or a colon net (a home colonic unit) because you don't want to go full speed ahead into an all raw diet and hit some dangerous walls without some help. So colonics bring up more issues for the people who are way into bowel cleansing than the people who are just starting out.

**People often ask how often they should wait between colonics. What would you tell them?**

If you're talking about the average adult in the raw food movement who's between twenty and fifty years old, in decent health, asymptomatic (meaning they have no obvious symptoms of illness), but knows he or she could be better, I always say, "Don't do any enemas or colonics if (a) your elimination is outstanding and (b) you truly, *truly* feel content, strong, energetic, centered, and full of life."

Once you've been on either a raw food diet or an almost raw food diet (or even a macrobiotic diet, following a month of eating tons of meat and bread) for a while and you start getting symptoms that you know are originating internally (breaking out, weakness, painful joints, bloating, fever, more menstrual pain than usual, and migraines are all common symptoms for people who jump into a raw food diet perhaps a little too quickly). If you are following the raw food diet and you are experiencing some combination of these symptoms, the cause is a full bowel. When you first get symptoms, call up a colonic therapist immediately because it's always about the bowel. If you want to try the enemas first, you can; but if you don't get rid of the symptom(s), or if you have a bowel evacuation like nothing you've ever seen, you need a colonic.

If you're in your twenties or thirties, very athletic, and in great shape, you might wonder why you feel this way. The more you follow the raw food diet, the deeper into the tissue the diet will go. It's at this point that you need help. What you have to remember is that the human bowel is meant by nature to pass yesterday's salad, not ten-year-old matter from 1995s steak and eggs. As you get into raw foods and this juicing game, you will loosen up your 1995 steak and eggs. Your body's not equipped to pass that on its own. That's what paralyzes the colon in raw food people. And if you are overweight or have a history of constipation (even though you may be asymptomatic), and you want to take on an all raw diet, I recommend you do a colonic a week for as long as you can. This is because a lot of people with bad bowels take on the Raw Food Detox Diet and only *think* they are eliminating really well. What they don't realize is that, while they are eliminating what they are putting in, they're also awakening the "demons" from years of constipation and bad eating—and they're not being eliminated.

Remember this: old matter comes out like hockey pucks; it does not come out thin and runny. So if you are only getting the latter from an enema or laxative, that is not a cleansing. That means the heavier matter is deep in the body and you must do a colonic. If instead of going on a raw food diet, you go on a macrobiotic diet or a Pritikin-style diet, that diet will be a lot less cleansing and you'll be able to get by on six or seven colonics a year. The more raw the diet, the more the colonic action comes into play.

### Why do people who eliminate every day still need colonics?

Well, there are two reasons. If you looked at the amount of food you put in your body and mashed it up in a pasta pot, you're not getting anything near that much out. But the second way to tell the state of your bowel is very easy. When you wake up in the morning after you go to the bathroom, suck in your midsection very deeply as you exhale. If you have a clean intestine that's not holding waste, your belly button should be almost kissing your spine. The midsection should be a cavern. It should almost look like you're starving to death. If you don't get that and all you can do is pull in a tiny bit, your intestine is full of matter and that's no good.

We all grew up eating pancakes, chicken sandwiches, Doritos, cheeseburgers. It doesn't matter what your elimination is; if you grew up eating "normal" American fare and you got into health in your twenties, thirties, fourties, or beyond, your body is impacted. It may not be as acutely impacted as someone who's less athletic, or who was born less genetically gifted, but it is impacted. *No one*, and you can take this to the bank, passes even 60 percent of the average standard American diet. Just because you are asymptomatic does not mean you are healthy. If you're an adult who is taking on a raw food diet, but on a twenty-year foundation of mainstream food, the time will come when you'll get extremely symptomatic and must do something with your bowel. Again, try enemas. If that works, keep doing them, but if you're only getting a leaky, runny release, try colonics.

**What is meant by *impaction?* How is it that someone who is very thin can have a lot of impaction and waste matter in his or her body?**

Fruits and vegetables are human food. Everything else isn't (other than breast milk). The degree to which certain foods are ideal for human consumption varies. In other words, sunflower seeds obviously are a lot closer to ideal than white bread. Now when you look at all the white bread, beef, and nonfoods that make up the standard American diet, that matter (again, to varying degrees) will stick in the intestinal track from the very first bite because it wasn't supposed to be put there in the first place. Now someone who is a marathon runner or gifted with a strong bowel may be able to pass a large quantity of it, but no one can pass 100 percent of a square peg through a round hole.

As the years pass, the body temperature, being 98.6°F, bakes the water out of the waste and it gets impacted into the bowel tissue. Here's a perfect analogy: picture a big puffy sponge that you'd use to wash or wax a car. Dip that in a bucketful of liquidy mud and swish it around in there until the whole sponge is full of mud. Then put it out in the sun in an Arizona desert for a day. Now we have a mud-filled, sun-baked sponge. That impacted sponge is analogous to the human intestine. An impacted intestine is the result of all the matter accumulated from consuming nonhuman food since birth. That matter is lodged in the cells, causing pimples, body odor, and all the other sicknesses and disorders that people deal with every day.

Now, even though certain people (especially if their diet is high in protein, and if their lineage and heritage are not given to obesity) may not blow up, this matter is still impacting their intestines like cement. This is why skinniness should never be equated with health. People may not show weight, but the toxicity is lining their organs like hockey puck rubber, their cholesterol count can be up into the 300's, and [they] probably have high blood pressure. Someone with that type of skinny body often will die of cancer earlier than an obese person because, in the latter case, the body is at least storing the toxicity away from the organs in the fat. That's why we can see very overweight people live to fifty and sixty before they eventually break down from their poison. But a lot of skinny people don't have the capacity to store the waste as fat, so it stays in the organs. These are the people whom we often see break down in their twenties, thirties, and fourties. So while it is true that everyone who is overweight is unhealthy, this does not mean that everyone who is skinny is healthy.

**Why isn't one colonic enough?**

Let's assume you've lived for thirties years on standard American fare. Suppose one colonic can remove a month of the residue of food that's stuck in your body like glue (and remember every meal that you've put in your body since birth that is not a fruit or a vegetable is partially stuck in the body like cement). Now let's suppose a colonic can remove a month's worth of matter—and that's a great colonic. Think about what you could eat in a day as a fifteen-year-old. Multiply that by thirty and you get a monstrous amount of impaction. If a colonic can remove one month's worth of eating and there are twelve months in a year, just do the math.

Anyone who thinks one colonic can take care of a lifetime of impaction . . . well, its like saying to Itzhak Perlman, the great violin player, "Itzhak, I took one violin lesson! When do I get to play the Met?" This whole life is a continuum. We learn as we cleanse, and we learn from our cleansing responses. We learn from the higher levels of energy, from the emotional releases that are coming. All of this is a long, beautiful journey. People need to let go of the medical paradigm that one colonic should fix you the same way one surgery should fix you. It didn't take ten minutes to create an impacted bowel.

### What are the different types of waste matter?

There are three different types of waste contained in the bowel. The matter that you put in your body over the last four to five days that hasn't quite left is *normal waste matter*. Matter going back a month or two or three, where it hasn't embedded itself yet in the intestines, that's called *putrefactive matter*. That is the matter that "stinks awfully." When you get into cleansing, you'll notice that what leaves your body is vile. That's putrefaction. However, the real deal is the *post-putrefaction*. That's matter that has been lodged in the body for so long it has turned into a gray, white, or black hard rubberlike substance that lines the organs like a hockey puck. When this matter leaves the body, which takes years of work, it has no smell. The only way to remove post-putrefaction from the body is through vegetable juice fasting (not water fasting) with colonics or the use of psyllium, bentonite, and certain herbs.

### How do you recommend psyllium be used?

Psyllium seed, in my opinion, should only be used by those in the best of health. It's a means for the person who is really pushing the cleansing to the final level. Psyllium seed is a plant which, when mixed with water and hits the large intestine, absorbs ten times its weight in waste off the intestinal wall. This sounds great, but most people's bodies are not equipped to pass this matter. It's too much, and it's too old. Now certain, very strong people who are just starting out can take psyllium and get some great results because it shocks the system. But as they get deeper into the use of psyllium and bentonite (liquid volcanic ash clay that drains toxicity from the other organs, not just the colon), which is an outstanding combination—they typically, and ironically, end up not being able to pass anything. This is because they are suffering from their success. The psyllium and bentonite are now attacking the oldest and deepest matter, and they need help. So I always tell people, when they start attacking the post-putrefactive matter, that no one should take this on until they've invested at least two good years in a really clean, vegan diet (70-percent raw) with a lot of bowel cleansing. You don't go straight from normal American fare to a lot of psyllium and bentonite. It's like asking a 300-pound man to run a marathon.

Anything you eat today that is not a water-containing fruit or vegetable is next month's putrefaction, and next year's post-putrefaction. That's what psyllium is about. It is the quickest way to get to this post-putrefaction. But only people who have been cleansing for a while or are in extremely good shape should use it.

**The question of transit times comes up frequently among raw foodists. Do you want to address how long foods take to move through the stomach and be eliminated by the body?**

Transit times are important because they guide how food should be eaten during the day. Stomach transit is the most important element in planning the diet. Intestinal transit is the most important element in gearing your results. Stomach transit times are the following: fruits on an empty stomach in a clean body or a moderately clean body can leave the system in thirty minutes. This does not count dried fruits, which take three hours. Salads (raw vegetables sprinkled with olive oil) take 1.5 to 2.5 hours, depending on the individual (the cleaner and more active the individual, the more rapid the transit through the stomach). Vegetables mix very well with grains or proteins, so it would be a good idea to eat a salad followed by a grain or a protein. But once that grain or protein enters the stomach, a minimum of four hours for the grain meal and a minimum of five hours for the protein is needed. If you're eating a mixture of grain and protein like, say, sushi, you should not eat until the following day because that meal will move so slowly through the stomach that whatever you put in it later on will ferment and turn to poison. If you keep transit times in mind, you will not ferment and trap your stomach. The quicker food gets through the stomach, the quicker it gets to the bowel, and the quicker it exits the bowel.

In terms of intestinal transit time, someone just eating fruit will see it pass about eleven hours later. Salads take about twelve to thirteen hours, and so on. But if everything's running into one another, you might as well be eating cheeseburgers!

**Raw foodists can become frustrated with the concept of sprouting their own nuts and seeds. Why is this often unnecessary?**

In the process of soaking nuts and seeds, germination occurs, which means that the dense proteins will be released. Once the nuts germinate, the body can break them down much, much easier because the alkalinity increases. This helps to remove density. There's a catch, though. While I don't discourage people from sprouting, I don't encourage it either—for two reasons.

First, any nut or seed that is not completely whole is incapable of germinating during the soaking process. When you see little chips of white, for example, on a raw almond, that nut will not germinate. So you're just left with a soaking wet almond. If a sunflower seed is chipped, it's unsoakable. Because of this factor and because of the time element involved, I don't really encourage people to do it. If we water up proteins that are ungerminated we are actually hindering the digestion of proteins. So if you have a bunch of raw almonds with chips in them and you soak them, you're not germinating them; you're just getting wet protein, and wet protein doesn't digest well. People are trying to do something for their own good, and all they wind up doing is getting bloated and gassy.

The other reason I don't encourage it is that once nuts are soaked, they don't taste as good—and this diet is difficult enough for a lot of people at the beginning, and we always want to keep the memory of what we were doing previously. If six months ago you were eating cheeseburgers, focaccia, and fish & chips, your body is in no way, shape, or form going to look at a raw almond as toxic. There's no reason to hit the level of perfection. Granted a perfect group of almonds that is soaked and blended is a little easier on the body. But if we don't like the taste of the food—if it seems bland—we should happily eat raw, crunchy, unsoaked almonds. It's still very high up the food chain, even though it isn't perfect.

So if you found that previously nuts and seeds didn't digest well, and the soaking and blending helps, do it. But be aware that foods like almonds, brazil nuts, and hazelnuts are often chipped, exposing their middle, which makes them poor candidates for soaking. This soaking business is for two types of people: the very enthusiastic, who have a lot of time on their hands, and the very ill whose ability to break down proteins and fats has become so compromised that they need to soak the food.

**People often associate raw foods with gassiness and believe that they cannot eat raw foods because it makes them uncomfortable in this way. What would you say to them?**
Basically that's like the scene in the exorcist when the priest puts holy water on the kid who's possessed by the devil, and the devil starts screaming and screaming. You're putting something very good on something very bad. When the average American raised on bad food with a lineage of bad eaters puts cleansing raw food in the body, the body's initial response is this awakening of poisons. This is interpreted as gassiness and cramps. In order to begin the cleansing process, you must endure these things.

But on the other hand, because so many Americans experience this symptom, we must understand the importance of transition. So what I would do with anyone who's complaining about that is have them drink an 8-ounce vegetable juice once a day, and then have them eat a baby blended salad (1 cucumber, ½ a bell pepper, 1 stick of celery, and 2 leaves of lettuce). They should also have about 5 tablespoons of this mixture before each meal, followed by their cooked vegetables, fish, rice, or whatever they choose after the blended salad. That little bit of raw food will not give them gas and bloating. After two months of this, they can increase their raw intake and reduce their cooked intake. But I believe that to pull a person off the street and not acknowledge their complaint of gassiness is a mistake that a lot of raw food people make. They say, "That's okay. You're just adjusting." But a person in that much discomfort is in such an acidic, nonoxygenated state that he or she needs to go slowly, include lots of cooked food, and not be egotistical or dogmatic.

**The concept that health begins in the colon is so intriguing. It always amazes people to know that the root of their headaches and joint problems are usually in the colon. Would you speak to this?**

That's a very good point. People always ask me questions like, "How can cleansing the colon clear the skin?" Think of the meridian concept (which is the basis for acupuncture, shiatsu, and reflexology) that there are literally energy passages running through the body like harp strings that carry energy and oxygen throughout the individual. Now what the acupuncturist will tell you is that various "harp strings," after years of wrong living, will get little clogs on them. Picture, if you will, gluing a jaw breaker or a golf ball to a harp string. If you then pluck that particular harp string, you're not going to get any sound because the ball blocks the passage of energy through that string. What acupuncture and shiatsu do is, by shaking the energy passages (acupuncture uses a needle, and shiatsu uses pressure points), try to dissolve the blockage so that it will pass through the blood, and out the bowel, the bladder, and the skin.

Now that worked in ancient times because people weren't that toxic. But nowadays, because the size and depth of the blockage is so deep, the subtly of acupuncture and shiatsu will not remove the matter. That's where the colonic/enema come in. Now getting back to the question, you understand that when you pluck a harp string that's clear, the entire string will radiate sound and movement—not just the part you pluck. And now that you understand that there are harp strings running through the body, the meridian concept becomes clear; meridians pass from the toes (where reflexology works the feet) up into the head and throughout the body in an elliptical shape.

The right-hand corner of the intestines (the secum) connects through the meridians that connect to the skull. The left corner of the intestines connect to the meridians that connect to the lower back and elsewhere. The transverse colon that runs from the right rib cage to the left rib cage connect to various other organs. Ergo, when we get clogged up in the bowel, we are stopping the flow of energy through the harp strings such that areas literally two feet away from the bowel are affected—the same way that a harp string with a golf ball attached to the middle of it, renders the whole string useless. When we empty specific parts of the bowel, the meridians that connect to that part have been freed and now are capable of making sound and vibrations again. That's why, when people empty their bowels, they feel their ankle, neck, and back pains go away. They are opening up their center to allow clear meridians to carry energy.

The body is more interested in its vital internal organs than in the skin, hair, and bones because we can live with slightly damaged hair, skin, or bones; but if our internal organs are damaged, we're in big trouble. What the system will do is push toxicity from the internal organs through the skin to save the organs. If you are helping the body with a cleansing diet, enemas, and colonics, there will be no matter to push through the skin—so your skin will become clear. That's why people who get into the cleansing lifestyle will get a lot of positive commentary about their skin.

# A CLOSING NOTE

My gratitude for this detoxifying lifestyle is beyond words. It has made my world richer in countless ways. Although nourishing the body with beautiful food is central to my life, this dieting lifestyle has actually liberated me from obsessions with food and body image. Now that my body always feels terrific and youthful, I never worry about putting on weight or live in fear of degenerative and chronic diseases. Nor do I worry anymore about what might happen to my body if I had another kid, or how I am going to feel in a bathing suit.

When I was much younger, I stressed about these things and frequently wondered, "If I feel this way now, how in the world am I going to feel about my body at thirty, forty, or fifty? It's all downhill from here." That was a torturous mindset that has no place in my current life because I have reclaimed the body and health that are my birthright. The proof is in the way I feel and what I see in the mirror. I am in no way out of the ordinary. My clients and I don't have some special, exclusive gene that makes the Raw Food Detox Diet work. We are just like you. And we are here to cheer you on because we know that you can—and will—reach your greatest health and beauty goals!

Here's to your body bliss!
*Natalia Rose*

## APPENDICES

## RECOMMENDED COLON THERAPISTS

**Chakra 17 West**
Portland, Oregon
503-493-9656
www.chakra17.com

**Chakra 17 East**
401 East Thirty-fourth Street
New York, New York
212-679-6576
www.chakra17.com

**Gil Jacobs**
528 Fifth Street
New York, New York
212-254-5279

**Prana Brooklyn**
Contact: Donna Perrone
825 Caton Avenue
Brooklyn, New York
646-435-7277

**For a trained gravity method colon therapist in your area, contact:**
**The Wood Hygienic Institute**
Kissimmee, Florida
407-933-0009

## RECOMMENDED DETOXIFICATION PRODUCTS

You may find all of the following detoxification products via the High Vibe Health & Healing website: www.highvibe.com/raw or call 212-277-6645. High Vibe carries a vast range of the highest quality raw food products available in the world, and is a one-stop shop for all items related to the raw food lifestyle. They ship products both nationwide and internationally. This means you can enjoy the best selection of pre-packaged raw food treats from the leading raw bakeries. After years of taste testing, I have come up with this list of my favorite brands.

## NATALIA'S FAVORITE RAW TREATS

**Blessing's:** Raweos (raw Oreos), teriyaki chips, coconut cookies, raw granola bars, and much more!

**Lydia's Organics:** raw crackers, dehydrated breads, raw granola (their grainless apple granola is the best I've ever had!)

**Didi's:** lemon-crunch balls, raw pies

**The Raw Bakery:** raw brownies

**Glaser Farms:** date-nut balls, golden flax seed crackers

**Living Nutz:** teriyaki and chili-flavored raw nuts (you'll swear they are roasted!)

**Good Stuff by Mom & Me:** raw breads and crackers, raw pecan pie bars, raw fig bars, and much more!

**Lara bars:** raw snack bars in many different flavors, including cherry, apple, chocolate, cashew, and cookie dough (Lara bars are also carried at many Whole Foods Markets)

For your convenience you can also find links to these products directly at my website, therawfooddetoxdiet.com along with a free copy of my newsletter.

Needak Rebounder
K-Tec Champ HP blender
Breville Fountain Juicer
Infrared Sauna
Yerba Prima Body Brush
Cara Enema Bag
Spiralizer
Mandoline

# RAW RESTAURANTS AND SHOPS NATIONWIDE

The following shops and restaurants are listed alphabetically by state. Please note that there are also many excellent health food stores (such as Whole Foods and Wild Oats) in almost every city in the country, where you should be able to find most of the transition foods (other than raw specialty items) that I've listed in this book.

## Alabama
**Golden Temple**
1901 Eleventh Avenue South
Birmingham, AL
205-933-6933

## Alaska
**Enzyme Express**
1330 East Huffman Road
Anchorage, AK
907-345-2330

## Arizona
**Tree of Life Spa & Restaurant**
Patagonia, AZ
520-394-2520
www.treeoflife.nu

## California
**Au Lac**
16563 Brookhurst Street
Fountain Valley, CA
714-418-0658
www.aulac.com

**Beverly Hills Juice Club**
8382 Beverly Boulevard
Los Angeles, CA
213-655-8300
Serves 100-percent organic juices, smoothies, and sushi rolls

**Inn of the Seventh Ray**
128 Old Topanga Canyon Road
Topanga, CA
310-455-1311
This high-end restaurant serves cooked food as well as a raw dish every night.

**Juliano's**
609 Broadway
Santa Monica, CA
310-587-1552

**Raw Energy Organic Juice Cafe**
2050 Addison
Berkeley, CA
510-665-9464

## Florida
**Dining in the Raw**
800 Olivia Street
Key West, FL
305-295-2600
Serves macrobiotic, vegan, and raw foods

**Living Greens**
205 McLeod Street
Merritt Island, FL
321-454-2268

**Suzanne's Vegetarian Bistro**
7251 Biscayne Boulevard
Miami, FL
305-758-5859

## Hawaii
**Raw Experience**
42 Baldwin Avenue
Paia, HI
808-579-9729

## Idaho
**Akasha Organics**
106 North Main
Ketchum, ID
208-726-5425
Serves smoothies, fresh nut milks, juices, raw salads, raw pizza, and dehydrated foods

## Illinois
**Karyn's Fresh Corner**
3351 North Lincoln Avenue
Chicago, IL
773-296-6990

## Massachusetts
**Organic Garden**
294 Cabot Street
Beverly, MA
978-922-0004

## Nevada

### Go Raw Cafe and Juice Bar
2910 Lakes Town Center
Las Vegas, NV
702-254-5382

## New York

### Caravan of Dreams
405 East Sixth Street
New York, NY
212-254-1613

### Health Nuts
1208 Second Avenue
New York, NY
212-593-0116
While there are many Health Nuts stores in Manhattan, this location has an excellent raw foods section!

### High Vibe Health & Healing
315 East Third Street
New York, NY
212-777-6645
www.highvibe.com

### Integral Yoga Natural Foods
229 West Thirteenth Street
New York, NY
212-243-2642

### Organic Avenue
23 Ludlow Street
New York, NY
212-334-4593
www.organicavenue.com

**Prana Natural Foods**
125 First Avenue
New York, NY
212-982-7306

**Pure Food & Wine**
54 Irving Place
New York, NY
212-477-1010
www.purefoodandwine.com

**Quintessence (three locations in Manhattan)**
263 East Tenth Street
New York, NY
646-654-1823

566 Amsterdam Avenue
New York, NY
212-501-9700

353 East Seventy-eighth Street
New York, NY
212-734-0888
www.raw-q.com

**The Sweet Dreams Company**
www.thesweetdreamscompany.com
They make sumptuous raw brownies!

**Urban Organics**
240 Sixth Street
Brooklyn, NY 11215
718-499-4321
E-mail: info@urbanorganic.com

## Oregon
**Well Springs Garden Cafe**
2253 Highway 99
Jackson Hot Springs
Ashland, OR
541-488-6486

## Pennsylvania
**Arnold's Way**
319 West Main Street, Store #4
Lansdale, PA
215-361-0116

## Washington, D.C.
**Everlasting Life**
2928 Georgia Avenue, NW
Washington, DC
202-232-1700

## West Virginia
**Healthy Harvest**
309 N. Court Street
Fayetteville, WV
304-574-1788

# BIBLIOGRAPHY

1. www.nof.org Website of the National Osteoporosis Foundation
2. www.european-vegetarian.org Website for the European Vegetarian Union
3. www.nexusmagazine.com Website of *Nexus Magazine*
4. www.all-creatures.org Online resource for a peaceable relationship between humans, animals, and the environment
5. Kulvinskas, Viktoras. *Survival into the 21st Century*. Fairfield, Iowa: 21st Century Publishing, 1975.
6. www.house.gov Website of the United States House of Representatives
7. www.betterhealthlchannel.com Informative website about healthful living

Baird, Lori. *The Complete Book of Raw Food*. New York, NY: Healthy Living Books, 2004.

Brotman, Juliano. *Raw: The Uncookbook*. New York, NY; HarperCollins, 1999.

Cole, Candia Lea. *Not Milk . . . Nut Milks*. Santa Barbara, CA: Woodbridge Press, 1997.

Cousins, Gabriel. *Conscious Eating*. Berkley, CA: North Atlantic Books, 2000.

Cousins, Gabriel. *Spiritual Nutrition & The Rainbow Diet*. Boulder, CO: Cassandra Press, 1986.

Diamond, Harvey and Marilyn Diamond. *Fit for Life*. New York: Warner Books, 1985.

Ehret, Arnold. *The Mucousless Diet and Healing System*. New York, NY: Benedict Lust Publications, 2002.

Ehret, Arnold. *Rational Fasting*. New York, NY: Benedict Lust Publications, 1971.

Gerber, Richard. *Vibrational Medicine*. Rochester, VT: Bear & Company, 2001.

Howell, Edward. *Enzyme Nutrition, The Food Enzyme Concept*. New Jersey: Avery Publishing Group, 1985.

Kulvinskas, Viktoras. *Survival into the 21st Century*. Fairfield, Iowa: 21st Century Publishing, 1975.

Meyerowitz, Steve. *Food Combining and Digestion*. Great Barrington, MA: Sproutman Publications, 1996.

Pottenger, Francis M. *Pottenger's Cats: A Study in Nutrition*. San Diego, CA: Price Pottenger Nutritional Foundation Inc., 1995.

Shelton, Herbert. *Food Combining Made Easy*. San Antonio, TX: Willow Publishing, Inc., 1940.

Shelton, Herbert. *Superior Nutrition*. San Antonio, TX: Willow Publishing, Inc., 1987.

Trotter, Charlie and Roxanne Klein. *Raw* Berkley, CA: Ten Speed Press, 2003.

Walker, Norman. *Colon Health*. New York, NY: Pyramid Books, 1970.

Walker, Norman. *Fresh Fruits and Vegetable Juices*. Walker Press: Pyramid Books, 1970.

Walker, Norman. *The Vegetarian Guide to Diet & Salad*. Presscot, AZ: Norwalk Press, 1971.

Walker, Norman. *Raw Vegetable Juices*. New York, NY: Pyramid Books, 1972.

Wigmore, Ann. *The Hippocrates Diet*. Wayne, New Jersey: Avery Publishing Group, 1984.

## ABOUT THE AUTHOR

**NATALIA ROSE, CERTIFIED CLINICAL NUTRITIONIST
FOUNDER, THE RAW FOOD DETOX DIET (A.K.A. THE ROSE PROGRAM)**

Best known for her highly personalized detoxification diets, certified clinical nutritionist, Natalia Rose's cutting-edge nutritional practice grew out of her vision to bring the benefits of deep tissue cleansing and detoxification into the mainstream. In addition to founding The Raw Food Detox Diet, Natalia Rose also acts as the nutrition director for the Frédéric Fekkai Spa in Manhattan. She also acted as the nutrition director for the Elizabeth Arden Red Door Salon & Spa for three years. Natalia also teaches vegetarian cooking classes for the Learning Annex. She has had the unique opportunity to work with some of the world's most body-conscious men and women—clients who demand the best results when it comes to perfecting their bodies. She advises models, actresses, media personalities, and social doyens whose careers and lifestyles hinge on looking young and beautiful.

Natalia also specializes in helping new mothers produce rich, superior-quality milk while regaining their best body ever and in getting even the most finicky child or infant to eat highly nutritious foods. She is also known for her fun and highly educational cooking sessions in private and group formats.

Natalia's media credits include the *New York Times*, NBC's *Live at Five*, National Public Radio's *On Point*, *First For Women*, and *Daily Candy*, and she was a regular contributor to the *Elizabeth Arden Red Door Newsletter* for three years.

Natalia firmly believes that anyone can enjoy vibrant health and lasting youthfulness—regardless of their age, old habits, or lifestyle—by making a few basic changes to his/her daily diet, and envisions a time when all Americans will learn how to stay youthful and heal themselves naturally.

Natalia received her BA at New York University and her certification in clinical nutrition at The Natural Healing Institute of Naturopathy. She lives in Manhattan with her husband and two children.

## FOR MORE INFORMATION, PLEASE CONTACT:

**The Raw Food Detox Diet**
Natalia Rose, CCN
917-887-3222
E-mail: Nr19@aol.com
Website: www.TheRawFoodDetoxDiet.com

# INDEX